THEY CAI

Freddie Odom

BUT THEY CAN'T EAT ME

FOREWORD

This book is dedicated to the hardworking men and women of the National Security Agency, because they already know everything printed in it. It's also dedicated to my family. Shortly before writing this, I lost my grandmother and my aunt, and I wanted to preserve whatever stories I could before it was too late.

It's dedicated to friends, to other mentors that I've had throughout the years, and to my greatest mentor, autism. Autism, ever since I first figured out that we were together, I've had to go back through my life story and sort out all of the mayhem that you've caused! (But, we're already married, so we might as well learn how to live well together.)

Disclaimer: If you are reading this and you are on the autism spectrum, I realize that you might also be on "the atheism spectrum." And I get it. Nevertheless, I've found it impossible to separate out the "God stuff," and have left these stories exactly as I perceived them when they happened. People of faith, Protestant, Jewish, Catholic,

Hindu and Buddhist, have been an important part of my life, and their stories deserve to be told, too.

For everyone who reads this book, I hope you enjoy it and I hope it meets your expectations, whatever they may be. If you do enjoy the book, I'd love to hear from you. If you hate the book...well, there are quite a few trolls on the Internet who would like to hear from you, too.

But that's a story for later.

CONTENTS

The Little House on The Pasture

"WHHHIZZZZZZZZZZZZZZ!!!"

"AAAAAAAGHHHHHHHHH!!!"

Such was the sound on the afternoon of March 16th, 1982, when Dr. Ralph Neal, a kind, goodhearted, aging country doctor helped me into the world. As he held me up, I returned the favor with a blast of urine. (I had been in the womb training to be a human for months, but bladder control hadn't been part of my training regiment. Besides, I was a little disoriented.) Fortunately, the Stork had dropped me into a hospital in the tiny town of Grove Hill, Alabama, where my grandmother worked as a nurse, and she knew exactly what to do.

After I left the hospital, I moved to my new home on Winn Road in Clarke County, along with my parents. My mother was a skinny woman with long, dark hair. My father was taller, also skinny as a rail, and was at once both bearded and balding. We lived in an old white house in the country (similar in design to an old sharecropper's house, though not quite as small. There was a well in the backyard. Across a barbed wire fence in the very back lay acres and acres of grassy pasture land. A horse whose owner no longer cared for him roamed wild throughout the fields, where there was also a natural spring.

In front of our house, across the road, there was even more expanse. There were only two neighboring households within walking distance (for a toddler, anyway.) In the first, there lived a family whose father had been in Vietnam; he suffered from flashbacks, and on some occasions ran outside screaming in the middle of the night. In the brick house next door, up a small hill, lived Lena Reeves. "Miss Lena," born in 1908, was a folksy, white-haired, determined old woman. Although we weren't actually relatives, I saw her as a grandparent and called her "Mee Maw." We would be constant companions for the next several years.

In part because I wanted to see Miss Lena so much, I often woke early and ran away from home. While my parents panicked, searched, and feared the worst, I would be sitting in Miss Lena's kitchen, eating biscuits and gravy (presumably squirrel gravy, she ate squirrels) before going into the next room to watch *Spider-Man and His Amazing Friends*. She must have had grandchildren at some point, because in the closet in her living room she had a box of toys which included my favorite metal bulldozer. She always called my parents and notified them if I was in her house, although on at least one occasion the escapee wasn't there: my panic-stricken parents found me under a tree near her house, feasting on fistfuls of rotten plums. As for the well behind our house, Daddy eventually sealed it up, because I loved the way it looked when I dropped all of his tools in it.

Miss Lena was tough, clearly having earned her way through the Great Depression. Her favorite meal consisted of squirrel, biscuits, and gravy. Whenever she did something that she thought might result in criticism, she responded with the curious phrase "Well, they can kill me, but they can't eat me!" To my mother, who was born in West Germany, who was seventeen when I was born, and who had probably spent more time living in Europe than Clarke County at that time, Miss Lena was a valuable mentor. Sometimes she would show up at the doorstep, telling Mama "Put on your good panties, we're going!" (There was no telling where they might actually be going.) She taught Mama canning and other survival/housekeeping skills that were useful on "the frontier" that was Southwest Alabama.

In fact, my community did feel like the frontier, and not only because everything was new to me. To a small boy, town seemed very far away. Some of the closest towns were Coffeeville (with about 300 residents), Grove Hill (pop. 1500) and Jackson (about 5,000.) The closest large towns were Selma, Alabama and Meridian, Mississippi, both over 90 miles away. If I wanted McDonald's (a real treat because they had Legos) it meant a trip 80 miles south to the old French port city of Mobile. The only large metropolitan city in our region was New Orleans, and I never went there until I was ten years old. Most of my childhood candy purchases came from a country store called Reeves Grocery.

The community that I lived in wasn't only physically remote, it was also culturally separate. When I was born, the number one song was "I Love Rock and Roll," and *Swamp Thing* was playing at the movies. The "decade of excess" was underway, complete with hair metal and break dancing. There was very little excess on Winn Road, however. As a young child, almost all of my role models were born before the age of television or even radio. When my mother watched episodes of Little House on the Prairie and I compared it to my own community, I couldn't tell much difference. In fact, when I first went to school in Jackson, I was sorely disappointed that it wasn't like the school on Little House. Maybe that was an early example of my perception being a little different, but maybe not. After all, most people from the Millennial generation probably can't remember dropping things down a well, or a tough old lady feeding them squirrel gravy for breakfast.

Family

When I was about five years old we moved into a brick house near the end of the road in Winn. This meant that I would see Miss Lena less; on the bright side I would be closer to my family. I had three grandparents and one great-grandparent still living in Clarke County. My father had eight siblings, my mother four. I had plenty of first cousins to play with (eventually twenty-four of them) and play we did!

It is nothing short of a miracle that I survived this period in my life, as my cousins and I rode a rusty, old wagon down the hill, fought in "wars" and played with guns. We ran and fell on piles of chestnut burrs (while not fatal, they could cause one to lose the will to live) and I crashed my cousin Moriya's bike into a briar patch. In one of the most dangerous events of my childhood, my cousin Amanda and I asked our parents for a bucket to collect "worms." The adults came outside to find us collecting a bed of baby rattlesnakes. There was no doubt about it, the outside world was dangerous. The fact that video games were invented probably saved our lives.

Visiting my extended family was a lot of fun. I visited my grandmother Margie, whom I called "Granny," often. She gave me bananas, let me read her medical books [red flag: five year olds do not usually enjoy medical books] and if I was lucky, she had a pot roast and some peas waiting for me. Like almost everyone in my family, Granny had a hard life, but you couldn't tell it from her attitude.

Granny was born around 1930; her mother died when she was young. Her father remarried, and the new stepmother put the children out on the street (during the Great Depression, no less) splitting them up to live with relatives in other towns. Eventually, she married a soldier and had nine children, but by the late 70s her husband was in poor health. In order to support the family, she had gone to college to become a nurse, at the ripe young age of fifty.

Granny's children, some of whom still lived at home, were David, Bill, Andy and Anita (the twins), Bettye, Fred, Marianne, Brett, and Angie. Out of them, I spent the most time at Bettye's house because she lived right across the road with her husband Johnny. Together they raised chickens, pigeons, dogs, and goats. Johnny, who always greeted me with "Hey little Fred!" had been paralyzed in work accident in recent years, when a line snapped and dropped the body of a dump truck on him. Now confined to a wheelchair, he took up the sport of racing and had all kinds of cars. He and Bettye had a pair of 1985 red-striped black Monte Carlos, but it seemed that his favorite vehicles were his El Caminos. His first racing car, a yellow El Camino called "The Yellow Jacket," sat in the garage.

My mother's parents, "Nanny" and "Paw-Paw" moved around a lot, but not too far. "Nanny" (who I actually also called Granny in spite of her wishes) didn't cook as much because she was from Michigan, apparently the land of undercooked vegetables. She had a habit of sighing a lot (which hurt my ears for some reason, I didn't know why) and my reaction to it got me into a lot of trouble. She didn't like to talk about her past (it turned out that she ran away from Michigan and was presumed dead) but she told me that she had only completed the sixth grade after her parents died in a car crash. Paw-Paw's favorite thing to talk about (and act upon) was fishing. I visited his mother Flaudie from time to time, too; like Miss Lena, she was full of ancient wisdom, and had a closet full of toys that I could play with.

I spent a lot of time with my aunts and uncles and made it to at least two of their weddings. The youngest was Angie, born when Granny was 43 years old. For numerous reasons including family hardship, Angie would be the first in the family to graduate from high school. For all of the holidays and good times I spent getting together with my aunts and uncles, I noticed that there was a particular day of the year in which all of the adults seemed sad: Independence Day. I soon found out the reason: on the evening of July 4th, 1979, Fred (my father) awoke to hear his dad stumbling and falling in the hallway, the victim of a serious heart attack. He tried in vain to revive him, but the doctors would later tell him that he couldn't have helped.

My grandfather Fred Eli Odom had served honorably during the Second World War. In the 1950s, he was sent as a state employee to Phenix City, Alabama (then under martial law) following the assassination of Albert Patterson. Later in life, during a time when the inner workings of clocks and watches were still tightly controlled by Swiss cartels, my grandfather figured out how they worked, subsequently opening a watch repair shop in Grove Hill. He wasn't without his faults: he would never overcome his two-pack-a-day cigarette habit, and he never told Daddy that he loved him before he died. Daddy blamed cigarettes for his father's death, and he had trouble understanding people who couldn't kick the habit; quitting smoking had been one of the easiest things he had ever done, he said, after watching his father die.

I never felt my grandfather's presence during my childhood, but I certainly felt his absence. Playing in Granny's yard with my cousins, I often saw the steel traps that had belonged to him, now covered in rust. I knew that my father had dropped out of school to work at a power plant because of his own father's failing health. I saw the impact that his death had on Daddy, too. During this time, he was "a hard man," angry at God and not necessarily known to run away from a fight.

About a year before my grandfather's death, my mother Sheri arrived in Clarke County. An "army brat" who had previously lived in West Germany, Italy, and Oklahoma, she had two sisters and a younger brother. As an outsider, she frequently got into trouble at school for violating sacred Southern traditions, like not referring to her teachers as "ma'am" or "sir."

It's safe to say that Mama had a fairly negative opinion of school at that time, and like almost everyone else I knew in Clarke County, she eventually dropped out. She met Daddy on a blind date in 1980, they married the same year, and the rest (as they say) is history.

Now we were all together, in the new brick house in Winn. My cousins came over to play, the rest of my family came over to visit. Life was good.

Life in Winn

Daddy packed his lunch every morning and went to work at a coal-fired power plant on the Tombigbee River. Promptly at 5:00 every evening, he came home tired and ready to eat. Having lived through the energy crisis of the late '70s, he was careful about how much gas he used, so he carpooled to work. One of the men with whom he carpooled had won over $200,000 from a contest on MTV, but subsequently wasted it all. Daddy was more careful. He had plans to work, save, and be a millionaire by the time he retired. He was in the union, the president of the local chapter at one time. When the union went on strike, Mama and I went to the power plant to visit the picket lines and take him something to eat.

Mama occasionally worked as a waitress (making my favorite gumbo at a restaurant called Shirley's) but mostly stayed home with me until I went to school. We watched a lot of TV (her favorite show was still *Little House on the Prairie*) but once we moved into the brick house we had new treat: a satellite dish! Unlike modern dishes (which receive communications from only one satellite) the older, "big ugly" C-band satellites rotated, allowing one to find preferred satellite signals. There were a lot of different channels to be found; some of them broadcast cartoons a day early, on Fridays. Although some channels were scrambled, a man came around the neighborhood installing modified decoder chips (reportedly at a cost of over a thousand dollars) to descramble the movie channels. This meant that when *Ghostbusters* was on Pay-per-View, I could watch it eight times in a row if I wanted to. (I hope the statute of limitations has expired on that, or my parents might kill me.)

Aunt Bettye had a satellite dish first. MTV was very popular among my parents' generation, and Aunt Bettye gave us a recording of videos from a day in 1986, including the world premiere of the Bangles' "Walk Like an Egyptian." My favorite videos were "Dude (Looks Like a Lady)" by Aerosmith, and "Fat" by Weird Al Yankovic, because I thought they were both pretty hilarious. Daddy was a *Guns n' Roses* fan.

Apart from MTV my favorite TV shows were *Masters of the Universe* and *Ghostbusters*. I watched the Ghostbusters movies obsessively, over and over again, while Masters of the Universe led to a fascination with swords and finally a plastic sword collection. One night, Daddy and I picked up a black man who was having car trouble and his granddaughter. Riding with me in our truck, the girl was so impressed with the glow of my *Thundercats* sword that I knew I was on to something that would make me very popular; unfortunately, Daddy soon disposed of all my swords because I had whacked him one too many times in the face.

I was a fan of *The Dukes of Hazzard* and collected the cars. I was also fascinated with Superman from an early age, thanks to *Super Friends* and *Superboy*. When I heard one time that Daddy was about to fight an unwelcome guest at Granny's house, I put on my red coat and started running up the driveway to stop the fight. At the car wash in Jackson the madness continued, as I leapt between huge vacuum cleaners, yelling "I'm flying! I'm flying."
Fortunately (lest I should have delusions that I was Super)

Miss Lena was there to put me in my place. She looked me in the eye and sternly replied, "No you're not, you're jumping!" And that was that.

There was no hope of watching any TV at all if a game was on. Daddy had a religion, and it was called basketball. He was a huge fan of Larry Bird, the "hick from French Lick." (I preferred Michael Jordan, leading to a divided house) Daddy was a basketball player himself, as the steam plant had its own team which competed against other plants and mills in the area.

One night while there was a game on television, I walked up and asked "Daddy, can I have an Apple Computer?" "Uh-huh," he replied, not understanding anything that had just happened. I ran excitedly into the back. "Daddy said I could have an Apple computer!!!" Mama was not amused. Nobody could afford an Apple computer; they cost over a thousand dollars!

Most of the time, I played outside by myself, walking around and kicking over the crawfish mud-houses that populated our yard. I had a bow and arrow that Daddy made me. Eventually he constructed a playhouse too, and Mama painted a Ghostbusters sign to hang on it. I had an old, black-and-brown dog named Buzzard that we found abandoned by the road, a black lab called Ruff, a pet rabbit who roamed freely in the garden, and the huge number of animals across the road at Bettye and Johnny's.

Being outside was also rife with dangers. For starters, there were all kinds of bugs in our yard (like fire ants) that were originally from South America, having come in through the Port of Mobile. I was bitten by a Brown Recluse, the second most poisonous spider in our region, and had to go to the hospital. Reptiles were a part of everyday life too; one day I kicked over a crawfish house only to find a snake inside. (Mama panicked and dispensed of it with an axe.) It seemed that everything outside was out to either bite me or sting me, so when we found a used Atari at a yard sale, the verdict was in: I would be staying inside.

Life in Winn was good, but there was also trouble brewing in Paradise. My parents were starting to have marital problems and were headed for divorce. My mother had two miscarriages after I was born and desperately wanted another child. My father had a flaring temper; even though he never hit my mother he did beat me a couple of times. My favorite cousins, Randall and Andy, were also having trouble at home. Eventually their parents would divorce and we wouldn't see each other anymore.

Nothing ever stays the same, but at least in our case that wasn't such a bad thing. Change was coming, and "God was on the move."

Standing at the Door and Knocking

No outside observer would have called my family religious. The one exception was my great-Uncle Noah Lee, who visited us from time to time. Noah Lee, who worked for UPS, was quite possibly the nicest person I ever met. When we discovered that I couldn't ride a bicycle, he said "It's all right. I didn't learn to ride a bicycle until I was thirteen."

Despite my family's lack of religiosity, we lived in a small, rural area out in the country, and we weren't immune to being invited to go to church with our neighbors. My first experiences with church were a bust. First, we visited Pilgrim's Rest Primitive Baptist Church with Miss Lena. At some point in the service, I thought it was over and went outside. There were other kids running, climbing, and playing around a big tree stump, so I stayed and joined in the fun. I had the time of my life! Then church ended, and I was in big trouble for skipping it.

We went to a church called Peniel twice. The first time, as a toddler, I reached up and caught a very annoying fly. That story became legend. The second time, at

Christmas, we had a bad experience because when I saw the Three Wise Men come into the room, I loudly protested the fact that they were giving away presents and I didn't get one. I may have made a scene.

Eventually my mother befriended a woman named Lisa who lived in a small trailer park in Jackson. I played there with her kids, watched music videos at her place, and in the process of watching videos I developed a crush on Mariah Carey (if I had known that someone from my generation would actually marry Mariah Carey, maybe I would have tried harder.)

At the edge of the trailer park, in a brick house, lived a man that everyone called "Brother Rivers." He was the pastor of the First Pentecostal Church in Jackson, and we soon started going there with Lisa. Brother Rivers was a Choctaw Indian and a fiery preacher. I thought that God probably looked a lot like him. Mama was serious about going to the Pentecostal church, but, she had very little religious background to work from. Once, I asked her to pray for me when I was sick. She became very upset, and with tears in her eyes, replied "I don't know how."

Soon Mama became pregnant again. She'd already had two miscarriages and worried a lot about losing a third child. Inspired by the story of Hannah in the Bible (who dedicated her son Samuel to God) she went forward in church, dedicating her unborn child to God. Several months later, my baby sister was born. Her name was Hannah.

My parents didn't have a lot of books, but there were two items on our main bookshelf: a set of Columbia Encyclopedias from the 1960s and a fluorescent red Illustrated Children's Bible. I read both of them, but I was especially interested in the Bible stories.

At one point, Daddy was staunchly opposed to the idea of our family going to church, and he did everything in his power to stop us. I had been reading stories from the red Bible and mentioned something to him about animal sacrifices. Daddy told me "You don't need to be reading that mess!" What I didn't know at the time, and it never occurred to me, was that the red Bible was his, a gift from a pastor in the years before his father died.

By the time I was in the third grade, my parents' views had diverged to the point that divorce was probably imminent, when my mother suddenly became very ill. She was placed in the Jackson Hospital, across the street from my school. Without Mama to help me get ready in the morning, kids made fun of the way that I was dressed. One of them said "Who dressed you this morning...your mama?" and with my literal way of communicating I replied "No...my Daddy did. Mama's in the hospital." (I think the kid felt pretty guilty after that. At least he shut up.)

After school, Daddy would walk me across the street to the hospital. Mama was in bad shape. She seemed to be dying of pneumonia, and had undergone painful spinal-tap procedures that left her unable to move. Daddy knew that she was on her deathbed. When we went home that night he decided to try something that he hadn't before: he prayed. When he came into the hospital the next morning, Mama was sitting up on the bed, brushing her hair.

The incident troubled Daddy and got him to thinking. He finally agreed that he would try going to church with us —but not the Pentecostal church! (He had visited there once. The environment, with everyone shouting and speaking in tongues and babbling about, was either too scary, too threatening, or both.) Instead, he agreed to visit Good Springs, a country church at the end of the road near Granny's house. My parents had been married there, and Good Springs was so small that even though they were Baptist and therefore believed in "dunking," they didn't have their own pool and held Baptism services at another church. Good Springs was safe and quiet. No one there would be speaking in tongues, the services would be short and closer to home, and nobody could try to baptize Daddy, either.

When we arrived at Good Springs on the first Sunday that we attempted to go to church as a family, we were greeted by the pastor, Don Stephens. Near the beginning of the worship service, Rev. Stephens announced that a visiting speaker (called an "evangelist") would be coming to the church for a week. He unrolled a poster promoting the event and announced the meeting times. When Daddy saw who was on the poster, he was stunned.

On the night that my father was to first meet my mother on a blind date, he was scheduled to work the night shift at the power plant. This was a serious emergency, of *Back to the Future* proportions. If Daddy couldn't get to the date, then he would also not make it to his wedding, and I would never be born!

To solve this problem, Daddy asked a coworker named Bill Bozeman to swap shifts with him. Bill, who was working the day shift, spent a lot of his evenings hanging out at nightclubs in Mobile, but he agreed to take the shift. Shortly after my parents' successful first date, Bill left work and disappeared.

Ten years later, my family was trying out church for the first time. The pastor unraveled a poster, revealing the speaker at the upcoming revival. His name was Bill Bozeman.

Daddy couldn't believe it! He decided to come back to church to see what his old friend was up to. It turned out that Bill's lifestyle of nightclubbing had been wearing him down for a long time. On the night that he traded shifts with Daddy, there were a couple of church deacons working at the plant. They had never discussed their faith with Daddy (maybe they knew his position already) but that night they did have a conversation with Bill. He listened to what they said, and a few nights later he walked by a theater playing a movie about the life of Jesus. He bought a ticket and went inside, and what he saw changed his life. He went home that night, opened a bag of Cheetos, poured a glass of Coke, opened a Bible and started reading. In the early hours of the morning, he hadn't touched the snack or the Coke, but he was still reading, with tears streaming down his face. From that moment forward, Bill Bozeman was a changed man. He left the Alabama Electric plant soon afterwards, eventually becoming a preacher. No one at work really knew what had happened to him or where he went.

Ten years later, Bill Bozeman stood in the front of Good Springs Baptist Church, less than a mile from our house. He preached there for a week, and Daddy attended every meeting. After church, he invited Bill to the house for more conversations. The difference that the Christian faith had made in Bill's life was obvious. By the end of the week, Daddy was ready for a change, too. He became a Christian.

The old Fred was gone. "All things were made new."

Good Springs and Good Friends

We began to settle into life at Good Springs. There were usually 30 to 40 people there, including several other children. The men (including me) often met for biscuits and "brotherhood meetings," and the church had a sunrise service every Easter (in which the churchgoers worshiped while watching the sun come up.) The singing was led by Mr. Sammy Finney, who was a great man, but hard of hearing and actually a little tone-deaf. (In fact, he was sometimes accused of "jailhouse singing" –being behind a few bars without the key.) Our songs came mostly from *The Country & Western Gospel Hymnal*, and my first public performance ever occurred at Good Springs, when I sang a gospel song called "Heavenly Sunrise."

Sammy took care of his wife Shirley, who didn't work, and his mother-in-law Nettie Nall, whom we all called "Mama Nett." Mama Nett, born around 1910, was the matriarch; it was rumored that her father had built Good Springs in the late 1800s. She fit an early pattern in my life, that of strong female influences born in the early 1900s.

These included Mama Nett and Miss Lena, but also Granny and my great-grandma Flaudie. While it wouldn't have been true to say that the region I was born in was matriarchal, by the time I met these women they were widows, and they ran the show.

When Daddy became a Christian, it was such a remarkable change that it nearly converted the entire family. Granny, along with several of my aunts, uncles, and cousins, started coming to Good Springs. Everyone in the family sang in church, especially Bettye. (Cassette tapes with background music, called "track tapes" or just "tracks," could be bought in town and used for special music.) We gathered at Granny's house after church for a pot roast, and every Sunday was like a joyous family reunion.

It wasn't meant to last, though. One night, in the church parking lot, Daddy told us that he felt called to be a preacher. He had been in talks with a Bible college, but in order to be admitted he would have to be both a high school graduate and a Christian for at least a year. Neither of my parents had graduated from high school, but they immediately began studying to take the GED. Daddy was so nervous about taking the GED that he had massive heartburn throughout the test and thought that he was having a heart attack. ("I thought my chest was going to bust," he later said.) I'll never forget the look of joy on my parent's faces when we went to the college in Thomasville to pick up their results. They both passed the test! Now that it was possible for Daddy to attend Bible college, an exciting new adventure lay ahead!

The next year was one of preparation. My parents worked to pay off any remaining debts, and my mother took a job working at McClain Hardware in Jackson. During the summer, we stayed with my Aunt Laurie and wandered all over town. At night, Laurie was the manager of the local movie theater, and I got to see good movies, like *Home Alone* and *Teenage Mutant Ninja Turtles II*, for free. When school was in, I rode home with Aunt Shannon, a teacher at my school, until my parents came home from work. By this time, Aunt Shannon was renting the little house in the country, next to Miss Lena, so I got to play in my old yard again.

Daddy also prepared by preaching at churches around Clarke County. He was very nervous at first and he still used a lot of very Cajun-sounding pronunciations. (I remember him calling the Woman at the Well a "woe-mun" the first time around.) Gradually, however, he got better and his confidence started to increase. He wasn't just a good preacher; he was a great preacher!

I prepared for the move by doing what I had always done: school. In fact, I had a pretty decent life at J.M. Gilmore Elementary. When I first went there, in Kindergarten, I was sorely disappointed that it was nothing like Little House on the Prairie. Instead, the school had many different rooms with many different teachers in it, and my class was outside in a portable trailer. When I arrived for the first time, I was asked to find my name and sit by it, and unfortunately, I couldn't find it; I had learned to read by sitting in my relatives' laps looking at newspaper headlines. I only knew capital letters!

To complicate matters, my teacher, Mrs. Sellers, nicknamed me "Freddy Kreuger." Whenever children thought of me, during my first year of school, I'm sure they thought of a scary demigod who could haunt their dreams and stab them, because they started calling me that, too. Kindergarten wasn't all bad, though. We were allowed to take naps, and in the afternoons we watched *The Three Stooges* or *Super Friends*, or whatever else happened to be on TBS.

As a fundraiser, the school sent us door-to-door selling chocolate. I didn't really understand the concept, so when they gave me a giant package of chocolate to take home, I took the only logical course of action: I ate it. It was so good, I also shared it with all of my friends on the bus, including a girl named Paige. I liked Paige a lot and decided that I would marry her someday soon. Fortunately it didn't happen, and I narrowly avoided a common Alabama stereotype. (As it turned out, Paige and I were related.)

In hindsight, it was evident pretty early on that I had motor coordination problems, but I usually came up with pretty good excuses for them. In kindergarten, I failed a test in which I was supposed to skip along to an old record of "Skip to My Lou." (I just ran past the record player and sat down.) I was also fond of Velcro shoes at the time, and I never really learned to tie my laces. Autism, or especially Asperger Syndrome, was basically unknown at the time; naturally, we just blamed the fact that I couldn't tie my shoes ON the fact that I liked Velcro. I was also "developmentally delayed" in learning to ride a bicycle. (We blamed that delay on the fact that we lived in the country and had a gravel driveway.) My parents bought Two Wheels for Grover, a book about the Sesame Street character learning to ride, to help with motivation. While I really was interested in riding a bike, I just couldn't. Besides, my great-uncle Noah Lee encouraged me by telling me that he didn't learn until he was thirteen, and that took some of the pressure off.

In the first grade, my teacher was Miss Andrews, a strict African-American woman who believed strongly in corporal punishment (if not also capital punishment.) She delivered spankings with a yardstick, and I was on the receiving end of at least two of them. (I didn't dare tell my parents about the yard-stickings either, for fear that I would get in even more trouble at home.) Another of Miss Andrews' early punishment practices was to make the children stand in the corner holding Sears catalogs over our heads, sometimes on one foot. "As their arms weaken, so too shall their wills weaken!" must have been the reasoning behind the practice. At any rate, when Sears announced a few years later that they would be discontinuing the Sears Catalog, there was much rejoicing!

My second grade teacher, Mrs. Tammy Breedlove, was very political. A traditional Southerner, she emphasized that Southern people were Democrats (though that view was rapidly changing at the time.) It was the end of the Cold War, and she taught us about the Berlin Wall, showed us pictures of people trying to cross it, and asked us to write letters to Mikhail Gorbechev. Inspired by the plot of *Superman IV*, I wrote Gorbechev a very nice letter asking him not to drop nuclear weapons on us.

I was interested in a girl in my class named Athena. One day, when Mrs. Breedlove stepped out of the classroom (Party time!) my classmates and I began running around and playing. We were having the time of our lives, really, when suddenly my Aunt Shannon walked by. "Look at what your son is doing!" Athena shouted, simultaneously selling me out and making a factually incorrect statement. Poor Athena. She may have been named after the goddess of wisdom, but it was never meant to be.

My teacher in third grade, Mrs. Lazenby, was by far my favorite teacher at Gilmore Elementary School. She had a piano in her classroom and used songs to help us memorize the states, multiplication tables, and more. In the mornings she read us stories, including stories from the Bible (a fact I liked very much, given the conflict in my family over those stories at the time.) She even taught us a song or two from Godspell. I actually cried the day that third grade was over, until my mother took me to town to see my teacher and take her a gift.

My best friend was named David. We shared a common love of wrestling, and of such superstars as Hulk Hogan, Macho Man Randy Savage, and Andre the Giant. I was obsessed with wrestling for quite a while, but one day I suddenly lost interest. In hindsight, my sudden obsession (then non-obsession) could have been something autism-related. At the time though, I reasoned that maybe hitting people over the heads with chairs wasn't such a Christian thing to be interested in anyway. At some point, our parents determined that David and I talked in class too much, so in the fourth grade we weren't allowed to sit near one another. It was a pretty grave situation, to say the least.

Meanwhile, moving day drew nearer. I stayed with Granny for a week while my parents went to Florida to search for a place to live. During this time, Granny did something that I had never known her to do before in her entire life: we went out to eat, at a restaurant. She ordered me cheeseburger pizza, in fact. This whole moving thing was turning out to be a lot more serious than I thought!

Before I left town to move to Florida, I had to let my girlfriend know. Yes, despite having been twice unsuccessful, I now had a girlfriend; I was head over heels in love with a girl in my class named Jessica Jordan. Jessica, whose father was a minister in Jackson, had shoulder-length blond hair, rosy cheeks, and an excellent singing voice. When she sang "Winter Wonderland" at the 1990 Christmas musical, I was captivated! (Sure, two other girls sang it with her, but as far as I was concerned she was the only girl in the third grade.) By the end of the fourth grade our relationship was doomed, and I needed to tell her that I was leaving town. There was only one problem: we had never actually spoken to one another!

I was very shy, and somehow Jessica and I had come to the understanding that we were an item without any actual direct communication. I gave her a card inviting her to my (probably Ninja Turtles-themed) birthday party once, but she didn't come. I gave her some Valentine cards too, also without speaking or receiving any kind of response. I finally received some affirmation when Jessica's dad Marty visited and spoke at Good Springs. Sitting in the row in front of me (but not too close!) she leaned over to one of her friends and whispered "That's my boyfriend!" It was pure magic. Super-hearing had its advantages, after all.

Jessica and I had been in the same class in the third grade, but the next year we were separated. As the end of the fourth grade drew near, I knew I had to tell her I was moving. In keeping with our communication style that had worked so well in the past, I needed some way to tell her without actually speaking to her. One day, as my class was going outside to recess, I saw her class approaching, and I knew that this would be my only chance. As her class marched past mine, I loudly chanted "I don't want to move to Flo-ri-da!" to one of my classmates. That got the message across, and a look of disappointment appeared on her face. She filed into Gilmore Elementary School, the rest of her class behind her, and the door slammed shut. My class marched onward to the playground, where I would soon be surrounded by kids running around, laughing and playing, oblivious to my inner gloom and despair. From that moment until my last day as an Alabamian, I never saw Jessica Jordan again.

Moving day arrived. I walked into my room, to see it one last time. It was completely empty, and its blue walls were bare. My mind was racing with memories. Daddy built a playhouse and fixed up an old go-cart for me at this house. In my mind, I replayed the first time I had driven that go-cart, crashing it directly into the pump house and throwing my sister out. My sister, about three years old, had landed perfectly on the grass, unharmed, saying "Whoah!" I ran away and hid under the bed, but eventually I got better at driving the cart. In fact, I had won every race against my sister's battery-powered Barbie car!

The go-cart and playhouse were staying behind. We had sold everything, and seemingly given up everything, so that Daddy could do what he felt God was calling him to do. After one final church service at Good Springs, and one final, difficult family reunion, we climbed into our car and headed for Florida, with everyone sobbing much of the way.

We came back to visit for New Year's Day 1993, beginning a twenty-year tradition of living at Granny's house while we were in town. We went around Jackson visiting my aunts and uncles' houses, and on their television sets I saw that Alabama was winning its first national football championship since the 1970s. It was a new era, and a spirit of optimism was in the air.

On the way out of town, we decided to pull into Miss Lena's driveway for a visit. We sat and talked for a while and had a good time, even if the visit was a little too short. Then we left and began the long trek back to Florida.

Two weeks later, Miss Lena died. Within the next year, she was followed by my great-grandmother Flaudie, Mama Nett, (the matriarch of Good Springs) and my great-Uncle Noah Lee. That old, noble, hardworking generation who had grown up before the era of television (or even rural electrification) lived through the Depression and two world wars, had seen the rise and fall of communism, and had taught me everything worth knowing, was now gone.

As a nurse who began working after age 50, Granny often tended to senior citizens who were on their deathbeds at Grove Hill Memorial Hospital.

"Is it time, Miss Margie?" they would ask.

"It is," she'd reply, and they would draw their last breaths.

Around the time we moved away, an 83-year-old man named Elige Steadham was on his deathbed. I didn't know it, but Mr. Steadham had performed my parents' wedding a decade earlier. He had been a minister in Clarke County for over forty years; in the course of his career he had been a great help to a lot of people. When he heard that my father had become a Christian, he followed the developments with great interest, and he had given Daddy (who until that point owned very few books) gifts from his personal library.

"I'm not worried about dying, Miss Margie," he said.

"You're not?" she asked.

"No…" he replied.

"…God has sent Fred."

God's Waiting Room

I grew up in an idyllic rural environment surrounded by family and elders, where people could make a decent living working on the river. Then, we sold everything and moved so that Daddy could attend Florida Baptist Theological College. In slang terms, Florida was known as "the place where people go to die."

We lived in Graceville, in a house on Ceiley Street that had formerly been a crackhouse. It was in the shape that one might expect a crackhouse to be in, too. There was a giant hole in the wall near the front door, among others. A soft, rotten spot in the floor caused Mama to have a nightmare about finding a dead body under the carpet. A broken pipe under the house leaked raw sewage onto the ground, and "Palmetto Bugs," a species of two-inch-long Florida cockroaches, infested the place. Walking outside at night, I could see the cockroach army congregated on manhole covers, drinking the condensation. We didn't have a telephone during that time, and received important calls from Jackson at our neighbor's house. Needless to say, when Aunt Shannon came to visit and help clean up the house, she cried a little.

Over time, our landlady agreed to buy materials so that Daddy could make repairs in the house. He put up sheetrock, plastered in the giant holes, painted, and planted a vegetable garden in the back. Thanks to that skillset, he got a part-time job doing maintenance work at the college. The majority of our family's income, however, came from my mother's new job at the Dollar General store. While my parents were working and going to school, my sister and I became "latchkey kids" and spent a lot of afternoons at home by ourselves. Thankfully, nobody ever knocked on the door asking for crack.

One good thing about Florida was that it was a melting pot, with all manner of retirees and even kids around. A family from the seminary, the Vosbrinks, lived next door to us, and we had the Collins girls across the street. The college had family housing too, and there were kids from all around the world there. One of my acquaintances was from South America, and my best friend on campus was a kid from New York named Joey, with whom I played a lot of Nintendo games. In fact, while I did play a lot of basketball, video gaming was the number one sport in my neighborhood. The consoles of anyone within biking distance were fair game, and it seemed like all of the kids in town traveled from house to house.

School was a different story. In Jackson, I had completed fourth grade and was headed for middle school the next year. In Florida, I found myself in elementary school again, because it lasted until fifth grade. If that wasn't enough of a disappointment, all of the kids in my neighborhood who were a year or two older were in an entirely different school.

I was also wearing glasses now, after a bout with Scarlet Fever (the doctor said it was unrelated.) While I had the occasional conflict with a student on the bus or something back home, I never had problems with bullies before. Now I was at a new school, and when I arrived as a shy outsider with giant glasses and no friends, I was stamped with a brand new label: "Nerd!" Nevertheless, one of my Sunday School teachers told me about the Sermon on the Mount, and I was determined not to hit back and to repay my classmates' "evil with good." Gradually, this started to pay off, and it resulted in a most unlikely friendship with a boy named Christian. Initially, Christian picked on me along with the other kids, but we quickly became best friends. It turned out that the bullies sometimes picked on him, too: his parents were immigrants and he was "Asian." (Christian's father was actually Austrian, but his mother was Malaysian, and they had moved to the area from Thailand.) Christian was a Buddhist, causing him to be constantly taunted by idiots with the phrase "Are you a Christian, Christian???"

Our friendship was somewhat unlikely, because while I lived in a crackhouse that had only recently become crackless, Christian lived in a mansion on the edge of town. I guess it would be fair to call it a "haunted mansion:" the previous residents, Robert and Kathryn McRae, had been murdered execution-style in the house in 1989. Their murder was an unsolved mystery. Robert McRae had been a former director of Gulf Power, and the murders followed both the disappearance of a graphic artist (scheduled to testify against Gulf Power in court) and the explosion of a whistleblowing senior vice-president's plane. As a result, any time I wanted to visit Christian's house I had to go through a security gate first. Whenever I spent the night there, Christian's older sister Susie tried to scare us by wandering the halls pretending to be a ghost.

I'm not sure that I ever really considered myself a child after leaving Alabama. My parents didn't make as much money as they used to, and I was conscious of that fact. I tried to take care of my sister and teach her the alphabet, reasoning that I had someone at home to help me learn to read when I started school. I rarely asked for things in the store because I knew we didn't have much money; instead, I did odd jobs for neighbors or sold some of my toys in a yard sale. I didn't have low self-esteem or anything because of it; it was just a fact of life. Besides, I knew that my parents had it much worse when they were kids.

Our budget for Christmas was a little smaller, and I noticed, but I didn't mind. One of the local churches actually came by and brought us a turkey. That first Christmas in Graceville, I received my prize possession: a bright red Swiss Army knife, just like the one my cousins had. (Actually, I got in big trouble that year for finding my Christmas present early.)

One of the best things about the holidays was being able to go back to Alabama and see everyone again. I even got to see the Christmas program at Good Springs! On one trip back there, Daddy was officially ordained as a Baptist minister. Brother Rivers came over from the Pentecostal Church to participate in the ceremony.

On another trip to Jackson, during the Arts & Crafts Festival, I walked by Jackson Middle School and stopped. There, sitting on the steps of the gym, was Jessica Jordan, the most beautiful creature I had ever known. She stopped mid-conversation and looked up, stunned. I smiled at her (we had never talked to each other, so why start now?) and I turned and walked away. I never saw her again.

Sometimes we had to make lightning trips to the hospital in Mobile. This was usually a good thing, like when my younger cousins were born. Other times we made the trip because of tragedy. One of my uncles put a shotgun in his mouth and attempted suicide; I didn't know why. Thankfully, he survived, but we weren't so lucky in the case of Granny's boyfriend "Doodlebug." Granny, not willing to take the chance of living with an alcoholic, told Doodlebug that she would never marry him unless he stopped drinking. Doodlebug killed himself. The deaths of the people that I knew back home weighed pretty heavily on me; I carried Doodlebug's wallet in my pocket for years.

Despite not really feeling like a child, I suppose I was one. I was able to find common ground with other children at my school. Christian and some of the boys in my class shared my common love of video games. I enjoyed mystery books, especially classics like *The Hardy Boys* and *Alfred Hitchcock and the Three Investigators*. (In fact, my teacher told me that I read TOO much, which was not something that I really expected a teacher to say.) In my class that first year, the biggest story of the year was the news of

Superman's death. We all became avid comic readers after that and began trading comics, just in time for the debut of the really fantastic X-Men cartoon. And we all loved The Karate Kid. A missionary came to our school once a week teaching karate lessons for $1. (Telling people that you learned karate from a missionary for a dollar can be a great conversation-starter, by the way.)

In religious life, we visited several places looking for a new church home. We went to one church two weeks in a row, only to hear two separate fund-raising pitches for the Cooperative Program. We went to another church for a while, but one of the members was a dirty old man who harassed the women. Finally, we started going to church with our neighbor Mike Vosbrink, who by now was pastoring a new church called Country Oaks Baptist Mission. The church met in a mobile home in a poverty-stricken area outside of Chipley, Florida, where at least one family was reported to be living in a school bus.

The Vosbrinks were great people. Mike was from the Miami area and had been on the Florida Highway Patrol before moving to become a pastor. His wife Pam went on a mission trip to Ecuador and brought back some Inca-style souvenirs for me. While playing video games one day, their son Jeff told me about a concept that I had never heard of before: the Rapture. That night, I had a strange dream. I was back in Winn, in the fellowship hall of Good Springs Baptist Church. There was a loud noise, and I started floating into the air. Unfortunately for me, I missed out on going to Heaven...because I got stuck on the ceiling!

One of the most embarrassing moments of my life involved Heather Vosbrink, who was slightly younger than me. One afternoon, as we were getting off of the school bus, Heather was loudly making fun of me about something. She had no idea that I had multiple issues with people making fun of me at the time, and before I even knew what I was doing I hauled off and hit her. She ran away crying, and I was horrified. According to my strict Southern upbringing by nearly Victorian-era women, hitting a girl was absolutely forbidden. I knew that I was the scum of the earth and I deserved to die.

I went inside the house to face certain doom, and when Daddy asked "What did you do today?" I confessed and told him the whole thing. I was grounded for a month. My parents blamed the karate lessons (despite my insistence that karate encouraged less violence) and I was never allowed to go back. Meanwhile, Daddy laughed at me, mocking the way that I'd told on myself, and I guess I deserved it. I never hit a girl again, that's for sure!

The Eleven-Year Old Protester

Eventually, the Vosbrinks moved back to south Florida and we moved into their house. In the absence of Mike, we started attending Harmony Baptist Mission, an interracial church that met in a storefront in Graceville. Maybe it was the church (I was taught that racism was a sin) or maybe it was the fact that I watched Gandhi in school, but I started to become a lot more socially conscious. In an empty lot at the end of our street, there was a graveyard where former slaves were buried. It was neglected and most of the graves were caved in. It was a constant reminder that while all men were created equal, some were more equal than others.

We were maybe a little less equal than others. With Mama's full-time job at the dollar store and daddy's part-time jobs, our family survived on about twelve thousand dollars a year. Uncle Noah Lee had given me a toy Dollar General truck when I was a boy, and I jokingly pointed at it and told my parents "We didn't know he was predicting our future!" Meanwhile, the "powers that were" in Graceville held a negative view of the seminary students and their families. ("They just think we're white trash," Mama explained, after enrolling Hannah in elementary school.)

In the sixth grade, I became the "teacher's pet" of an African American woman named Mrs. Douglas. To be completely honest, Mrs. Douglas was scary. She spent the first day of sixth grade yelling at us and telling us that she wasn't going to put up with our bad behavior. (Her scare tactics worked; I don't remember any behavior problems in her class all year.) Luckily for me, my first name was Douglas, and she insisted on calling me that. While Mrs. Douglas might have been very stone-faced and strict, she would quietly give me her "extra" books and candy sometimes. She chose me to do a presentation about Rosa Parks for the Parent/Teacher Association one night.

The assistant principal's daughter Angie either liked me or pretended to (I couldn't tell the difference) and one day, I arrived at school to find that several of my friends were skipping class to protest in front of the high school section of our school. Apparently, Graceville High School still had segregated proms, and an interracial couple had been refused entry by the principal. Angie's mother had publicly opposed the decision, and as a result she was to be moved to another school elsewhere in the county.

Today the students were protesting outside, chanting "Hell no, we won't go!!!" Various school officials were sent out to try to convince us to go back to class, but to no avail. After getting over my initial shock that the high schoolers were saying "hell," I joined the protest and just said "heck," despite the principal's threat that any student who skipped class would receive a grade of zero. We stayed outside for hours. The police stopped us from marching through town at one point, but since the local CBS station was filming the protest it remained peaceful and never got out of hand. I might have gotten six zeroes that day, but I was proud of my classmates and knew that we were doing the right thing.

Years later, I would teach sixth grade students, and my model for doing so was Mrs. Douglas (minus some of the yelling, of course.) Some of my students would complain that their work was too hard, but I couldn't relate. After all, when I was eleven years old, I was doing landscaping jobs in my neighborhood. I was trying to help raise my sister. And I was marching in the streets during my first political protest.

With a Little Help from My Friends

By now I had a core group of friends at school. Aside from Christian (who had moved from Thailand and lived in a mansion on the edge of town) there was Robert, who lived down the street. Robert's parents had divorced and remarried, so he had multiple sets of grandparents, and they bought him every kind of new experimental video game accessory. He had the usual Nintendo and Sega consoles, but he also got rarer things like the Sega CD or 32x models. While I had a Nintendo pistol to play Duck Hunt with, he had some kind of Nintendo bazooka. For fighting games, he even had a vest that vibrated whenever someone was punched by another player. We spent the most time at Robert's house, because he had all of the cool stuff.

I had friends outside of school, too. My dad had a friend from college named Mike, who had basically been a pool hustler for a living before becoming a Christian. His daughter Tiffany and I were friends. At the college, I played with a kid named Joey a lot, who mother was a New Yorker.

Hannah's best friend across the street, Jessi, had older sisters named Becky and Abby who were among my best friends.

One day, Abby invited me to First Baptist Church (my family usually avoided churches with "First" in the name; I thought they were "snooty.") to a new program called "True Love Waits." I said "Okay," and off I went.

It turned out that True Love Waits was about sex. I was extremely embarrassed to be there, especially when I saw Robert sitting across the room. I had already been through sex education at school in the fifth grade, and I 'd hated it too! Participants were given a sort of promise ring and asked to sign a pledge that stated:

"Believing that true love waits, I make a commitment to God, myself, my family, my friends, my future mate and my future children to be sexually abstinent from this day until the day I enter a biblical marriage relationship."

An abstinence education program was not out of the ordinary in Florida in the mid-1990s. (Apparently 2.5 million people went through the same program.) What was entirely special about True Love Waits, however, is that there was a soundtrack, and we were fortunate enough to receive a copy. The soundtrack was full of Christian pop songs, some of which were cautionary tales about people who had sex too early and faced the consequences. The first, and perhaps the campiest, song on the album was a rap song called "I Don't Want Your Sex For Now." It was catchy. And kitschy. I still jokingly sing it to my wife sometimes.

Having survived True Love Waits, Robert and I also drew comics and passed them around in class from time to time. We were constantly bombarded with drug advertisements on TV, so we thought it would be funny to base our comics on that idea. My comic strips were about the adventures of a superhero that lived on the planet Gas-X, while Robert's superhero strip was called Mylanta Man. The man from Gas-X looked kind of like Blue Beetle, while Mylanta Man was a long-haired, muscular hero who always held his hands behind his back (because Robert couldn't draw hands.) The comics industry was booming at the time, and the two of us agreed that we would open up a comics shop together as soon as we finished school.

Christian's family had a ranch in Cottondale, Florida. He and his sister Susie were accomplished equestrian show jumpers. I spent some time at the ranch, watching them practice and learning rudimentary horse skills. (These were very basic skills, like how to lead a horse, how to brush a horse, or how to not get kicked in the face by a horse.)

Two of my other friends at school were Robbie (who I thought liked the Power Rangers just a little too much) and Mark, whose cool dad took us to Panama City Beach during Spring Break. It was on that trip that I heard a Green Day song for the first time, and after that my musical tastes started to shift in a very punk rock direction (until the present day, really.) As Karate Kid fans, we all went together to see the premiere of The Next Karate Kid, and after we saw D2: The Mighty Ducks I became interested in street hockey, sometimes rollerblading for hours every afternoon.

There was a kid named Jeffrey in our class who, like me, was skinny and wore glasses. I noticed that he wasn't quite as unpopular as me, because he was the class clown. I made a mental note of the fact that jokes could decrease my suffering and began to practice comedy as a survival skill. I found out early on that if you're face to face with a guy who wants to fight you, and you make him laugh, you might live to see another day.

Every morning, we kicked off the day by watching Channel One News. For the uninitiated, Channel One was an advertising service that provided TV sets to schools as long as each school agreed to show their flagship program each morning. That program, Channel One News, consisted of about 60 percent Mountain Dew commercials, 20 percent something from the Ad Council, and 15 percent clips of Anderson Cooper dodging mortar shells.

One morning while Channel One was on, Jeffrey became very upset. Why? Was he concerned for the well-being of our hero Anderson Cooper? No! "Kurt Cobain is dead!" he exclaimed. Apparently Kurt Cobain was his older brother's hero. I had no idea who he was; during my last three years of not having cable, I had missed something very big.

I was interested in music, though. Christian was in the band (playing trombone, I think) along with most of my other friends, and I wanted to join. I went to an interest meeting in the sixth grade, but the band director said that the only position available was to learn the snare drum. I couldn't join because my family really couldn't afford a snare drum at the time, but I was invited to join the Junior Beta Club with my friends. This created the background for my first ever political campaign.

One of our classmates was the son of a mayor from Georgia, and the youth leader at the storefront church that I'd attended told me that he was elected student body president at his school, because all of the unpopular kids voted for him. That idea stuck with me, and I decided to try it out. I convinced Robbie to nominate me for Beta Club president. The election was held, and soon the results were in: In the first election of my life, I received zero votes.

I enjoyed my time in the Beta Club anyway, because we soon traveled to the state convention in Orlando and I had a great first experience in the city. Unfortunately, I discovered that I'd lost my wallet in the hotel. When I headed back to the elevator to look for it, the door opened, and behold! One of our advisors was holding the wallet in her hand. I was relieved! That is, until she opened her mouth and said "You'll have to give me a kiss first!" Our Beta Club advisor looked to be over fifty years old, but I did the deed and got my wallet back. It was my first kiss. I was horrified. I probably broke my True Love Waits pledge.

I began to excel in academic competitions, winning a first-place tri-county math trophy and eventually the school spelling bee. The editor from the local newspaper came to interview me about it, and he asked "How do you feel about winning the Spelling Bee?"

"I don't really care," I replied.

The next edition of the paper featured a picture of me, along with a caption that read something like "I am very honored to have received an award in this competition and will do my best as I represent the school in the countywide contest."

That liar! From then on, my friends and I would occasionally play ball in the empty lot behind the newspaper office. Whenever the reporter came out to get in his car, I would glare at him, silently judging him for misrepresenting what I said. Unfortunately, that would be the least of my worries, because this lying liar and I would meet again.

One afternoon, after a fun day of playing basketball with my dad and neighbors, I decided to ride my bike over to Robert's house. "He's not home," his mother said, but she told me where he was, and I decided to go and find him. When I stopped at the stop sign at Florida Highway 2, I had a bad feeling. I should have recognized the feeling; I'd had the same one in the fourth grade, during our class trip to the zoo in New Orleans when a car pulled out in front of us and wrecked the bus.

There were overgrown bushes around the stop sign at the edge of Highway 2, but I looked both ways and didn't see any oncoming traffic. I had just begun to cross the street, when suddenly I was struck by an oncoming car and knocked ten feet into the air!

When I awoke several minutes later, a crowd of people was standing around me. They told me not to move, but I told them I was fine. I walked over to pick up my bicycle, but it was crushed. Every inch of my body was in pain, but I ignored the onlookers again and started limping and trying to walk home. Then I collapsed onto the pavement.

I have no memory of the next three days, except for one image of my next-door neighbor, a police officer, standing over me in the emergency room. (Curiously, I have two different memories of how the accident happened, so one of them must be a dream or hallucination.)

Mama filled in the rest of the details later. She was at the Gulf Power office, paying our electric bill and talking to a friend who worked there, when she saw a crowd gathering down the street. She walked over to see what was going on, and there I was lying on the ground. She lost her composure, not only because I had been hurt, but also because one of the bystanders had placed a red towel under my head; she thought I was bleeding to death. At that point, the newspaper reporter walked by and snapped a picture of me lying on the pavement. "You're not going to put that in the newspaper, are you?" she asked, appalled. "No, I'm not" he promised, and walked away.

The woman who hit me declined to claim the accident on her insurance, because she worried that her rates might go up. If she had, her insurance coverage would have paid my medical bills. Instead, it took my parents years to pay off the debt from my few days in the hospital. (I felt pretty guilty about that.) The next day, on the front cover of the local newspaper, there was a picture of me lying bloody and unconscious in the street. Mama had a nervous breakdown. Some people were more equal than others.

My friends came to visit me in the hospital. When I returned to school, I was sore and had lost a little confidence. I had suffered a concussion, and wondered if I had brain damage. I think my grades started to slip a little, too. But I got "by with a little help from my friends."

As the year drew to a close, however, it was like a cue ball had struck my cluster of friends. We would soon be scattered all over the world. Daddy was almost finished with seminary and would be pastoring a church in Georgia. Christian was moving to Malaysia and I would lose track of him for at least ten years after that (until I found out that he was living in Alberta, Canada.) Robert was moving to Andalusia, Alabama, where his dad lived, and other kids were moving elsewhere throughout the Southeast. I couldn't particularly drive to Malaysia or Andalusia, so it was like a death sentence to me.

On the last day of school, the bell rang. When we got up to walk out of science class for the last time, Christian and I stopped, ran to one another, and embraced. As time passed on, I sent him some letters addressed to Kuala Lumpur, Malaysia, but I never got a response. Meanwhile, we loaded a U-Haul and headed to Georgia. As was my custom, I walked into my empty room one last time, looking for some closure.

In the 1980s, a film called *Stand By Me* was released. I saw it after I moved to Georgia, and it's not my favorite, but there is a quote at the beginning that has always stuck with me:

"I never had any friends later on like the ones I had when I was twelve.

--Jesus, does anyone?"

Vernon, Florida

Unbeknown to my friends at school, I had been secretly leading a double life. My dad, who worked several part-time jobs throughout college, was finally called to pastor his first church, Live Oak Baptist Church. It was located outside of Vernon, Florida (about 45 minutes away) in a community called New Hope, and it became my "home away from home."

What I didn't know at the time was that Vernon was famous. Well, sort of infamous. Vernon had been the subject of a cult film by Errol Morris called *Vernon, Florida*. "Why was it called Vernon, Florida?" you are probably not asking? Well, other than the obvious reason, Morris changed the name because he received death threats when he was going to name it Nub City.

Apparently Vernon was known during the late 1970s for a type of insurance fraud in which people would actually sever their own limbs in order to claim insurance money. Morris was given $2,000 to travel there and conduct interviews, but his life was soon threatened by people who feared that he would let their secret out and cause them to be jailed with no limbs.

Morris returned later and decided to focus on some of the eccentric people who lived there instead. There were lots of them to be found; as in much of Florida, there was a lot of rural poverty there, but there were also a lot of eccentric people who emigrated from somewhere else. The film featured several people who weren't native to Vernon, but the "star" of the show was a local turkey hunter named Henry Shipes, whom reviewers of the film called "religious" about turkey hunting. Henry's brother Murray was a member of our church, and I always thought he was a pretty smart fellow. In fact, I can personally attest to the fact that no one at Live Oak Baptist Church ever had nubs.

During the entire time that I knew the Shipes family, I never heard mention of any film. I later learned that it was a sore subject in town, and that a lot of people thought it was made to make fun of the people there. It probably was.

However they might have been portrayed on film, there were some really great people in the New Hope community, and some very interesting ones, too. Earl Evans, a retired Korean War veteran, lived there with his wife and grandson, and I spent a lot of time at their home. Despite being over 60 years old, Earl took so his grandson Earl III on motorcycle trips across the United States every summer.

Among the nicest people in New Hope was Andy Taylor, who hailed from Ohio and came to live in Vernon after retiring from the 82nd Airborne Division. His wife Rose wrote more encouraging letters and cards to people than anyone I've ever met (Daddy said she wrote so many letters that the post office gave her her own zip code.) Even after we no longer lived in Florida, she wrote to us for many years.

Because there was more than one worship service (morning and evening) we stayed in New Hope all day every Sunday. People often invited us over for lunch, and it's quite possible that I was in every house in that community at one time or another. When we weren't invited to someone's house in the afternoon, we stayed in a small room in the church that had a couple of old couches in it and a copy of The Serenity Prayer on the wall. On weekends and during the summer, Daddy took me "visiting," which meant going to visit church members, especially sick ones, or inviting people in the community who didn't go to church to join us.

Live Oak was a melting pot, mostly of old military veterans from around the U.S., but the occasional odd character, too. One of our church members' husbands was a New Age artist who believed in reincarnation. Another had a house completely decorated in ship's wheels (including coffee tables made from them.) There were little old ladies who sat at home watching Gaither (a gospel music group from Indiana) videos. A band of teenage brothers who lived in a trailer park with their father and "a bum" came to church without their parents. One couple at the church lived in Panama City Beach, where they managed a resort called The Dunes of Panama. We rang in

January 1, 1994 from the top-floor suite of the Dunes, watching the fireworks flare across the Gulf Coast!

Like my neighbors in Winn, there were many salt-of-the-earth people in New Hope who had lived through the Depression: when I stayed overnight at the Evans' house, I was only allowed to run about two inches of bathwater. (Conservation and frugality were embedded into that generation.) There were younger people, too. Daddy had a long-haired musician friend named Mark who often played at the college in Graceville, and he invited him to come and perform at Live Oak.

There was a younger couple in the church named Joe and Olinda Taylor who spent a lot of time with me, taking me to a rodeo and (most importantly) introducing me to the game Wolfenstein 3-D. (Joe was a CPA, so he was the first person I met to have a computer at home.) Joe and Olinda were unable to have children of their own, though they tried. When they finally succeeded, the baby only lived for six days. It was a catastrophic moment in the life of our church. While death is not final for Christians (and all of us believed that) the image of everyone standing outside, surrounded by Spanish moss, while Joe carried out a white, preemie-sized casket haunted me. I didn't go to funerals again for years.

There were a lot of funerals at Live Oak in the twenty years since, and sadly I missed all of them. Life goes on. Joe Taylor is now the Superintendent of schools in Washington County, Florida. And my dad's friend Mark, the long-haired musician who once played at our church? His name is Mark Hall, and he has sold over 5 million records as the lead singer of the group Casting Crowns. Few people have done that since Napster was invented. The truth is sometimes stranger than fiction.

A storm was brewing that would keep us from being in New Hope for much longer. Live Oak was a Baptist church, technically democratic and ruled by majority vote. In reality, however, whatever the secretary and her husband said ruled the day. If the secretary didn't like or agree with what Daddy said when he was preaching, then she would simply refuse to pay him. For a family of four living on an income from Dollar General and driving over 40 miles to church, that made life somewhat difficult.

Of course, there was a literal storm brewing, too...

Before the Flood

I awoke to the clap of thunder, louder than any I'd ever heard before, and stumbled into the hallway. The house was pitch-black, except for the unbearable brightness of the lightning outside. The wind was tearing through the house fiercely, and I called for my parents. They couldn't hear me over the sounds of the wind and thunder. Above, I heard the sound of the roof coming apart. It collapsed on me, and it was over.

I woke up again. The house was...still standing? I was alive! It had all been a dream (but I would never be able to relax and enjoy the sounds of a thunderstorm ever again!) The storm raging outside, however, was very real. The wind was howling, rushing along at 65 miles per hour.

Less than two weeks after the baby's funeral, on July 3rd, the first storm of the Atlantic hurricane season slammed into the Florida Panhandle with a fury. On the evening news, I saw people in Panama City and elsewhere boarding up their shops, anticipating serious wind damage. While people in Florida knew how to prepare for a hurricane, no one was prepared for Tropical Storm Alberto. Outside of our house, the storm gusted at up to 75 miles per hour and caused some significant damage around town. No worries; Atlantic storms tend to do that...what we didn't expect is that the storm simply wouldn't leave. It stalled, dumping floodwaters over the whole area.

The entire region eventually flooded, and I don't just mean Florida. The towns of Elba, Alabama and Montezuma, Georgia, both surrounded by levees, were completely inundated. In Georgia, the city of Macon was completely cut off by floodwaters, while the city of Americus recorded nearly 28 inches of rain.

At our home in Graceville, Florida, the streets were flooded but our house wasn't, save for a little water in the garage. The New Hope community where we went to church, however, was a different story. We had to cross a fairly high bridge in order to get to the church building; when we went to a prayer meeting a few days after the rain started, there was already violent, muddy water flowing just inches below the bridge. Many of the outlying areas around Vernon were populated by people who didn't have very much money. They tended to live in low-lying areas; their homes and possessions were washed out.

I was out of school for the summer, so I rode with Daddy to Vernon every day. We did some relief work, redelivering supplies from the Red Cross, but we mostly visited the homes of people in the area surrounding the church, so that Daddy could "strip out" their houses. The process went like this: when we walked into someone's home, we could see a "water line" on the walls indicating how high the water level had risen in the house (sometimes six feet or more, taller than me.) At the very least, the walls below that line had to be torn out, with all of the sheetrock, plywood, etc. removed. Meanwhile, the families bagged up their water-damaged possessions and clothing and stacked the bags outside.

Some of the children that I went to church with had to be rescued by boat. (It was also a terrible cultural loss, I might add; one of those children had an original "Pong" arcade in her house.) There were some long-haired teenage boys who lived in a trailer park by the river, who hitched a ride to church every week. The trailers were wiped out, and I never saw them again after the flood.

Daddy did, though.

One day he went to help the boys clean up and move out. He came back with tears in his eyes. One of the boys, named Jesse, had given Daddy his only possession that survived the flood: a lucky horseshoe. In the decade that followed, Daddy kept that rusty old horseshoe nailed to the wall in his office, a constant reminder of why he became a pastor.

Some of the people who lived around our church were made homeless by the flood. A few did what they could to help. But every organization can have its bad apples. One elderly man whose house was unaffected actually took the water that the National Guard put out for the flood victims. A few others stopped Daddy from using the church building as a shelter, saying that the people whose homes were flooded were "bums." As mentioned in a preceding paragraph, the church secretary even stopped paying Daddy if she didn't agree with his sermons (and that had no small effect, since our family was then living on about $3,000 per person, per year.) Eventually the pressure was simply too much.

Daddy resigned as the pastor of Live Oak Baptist Church. When the majority of the members found out why, they were "righteously indignated" and sacked the secretary for abusing her power (even though many of the church members were related to her.) A secretarial coup took place in which Joe Taylor (himself a Certified Public Accountant) took over.

It was too little, too late, however. On the last day that Daddy preached at Live Oak, I went into a room with him and told him that he was making a mistake, that God didn't want him to quit. The secretary, Mrs. Gertrude Weaver, had been around a while (having been born in the 1910s) and she was one of my Sunday school teachers. I thought that I could broker an agreement between them;

alas, it turns out that twelve year old boys are not great negotiators in such situations.

In later years, Daddy mused "Maybe I did leave too early," but who could blame him? In the span of about five months, I had been hospitalized after being hit by a car, he had to perform a funeral for a six-week-old infant, and after a catastrophic natural disaster hit the church, he made an 80-mile round trip every day to pick up the pieces, often without pay.

Hurricanes and floods like the one we experienced are sometimes called "Acts of God." I beg to differ. I'm much more fond of a slogan used by the Salvation Army: "Combating Natural Disasters with Acts of God." In the summer of 1994, I watched and worked as I saw Fred Odom performing Acts of God. It has been said that "great men are forged in fire," and that was true of my father.

As for me, it could be said that I was forged in flood.

Georgia Blues

I had a dog, a black lab named after Dennis the Menace's dog Ruff, who wandered up to our house when we lived in Alabama. He made the trek with us to Florida, where living in town didn't suit him as well. Now we were on the way to Georgia, and if leaving all of my best friends behind wasn't bad enough, Ruff was providing insult to injury, leaning over and slobbering all over me every time I tried to open my bag of lunch.

When we arrived in our new community, "Colomokee," there was a committee of neighbors waiting to help us unload the truck and unpack. The kids from our new church were there, and I quickly challenged them to a game of street hockey in the back of the moving van. (It would be my last time playing, too: while I previously rollerbladed for hours every afternoon, the bumpy country roads in Georgia weren't suitable for skating or skateboarding)

There was a pretty, curly-haired girl in the neighborhood named Summer, who officially became my first friend in Georgia. The point at which we actually became friends is uncertain, because in keeping with past tradition I was mostly too shy to talk to her. Nevertheless, a couple of weeks after we moved in I was invited to go with her to summer camp; since she was a farmer's daughter, we soon found ourselves on the way to Farm Safety Camp.

It's important to point out that at this point in my life, I had never really been exposed to modern farming. I say "modern farming," because I had been exposed to what anthropologists call "subsistence farming." Daddy grew most of what we ate when I was younger, and I spent a million hours of my childhood shelling peas, shucking corn, etc. We did almost everything by hand. Daddy called this "gardening," but that label might have been questionable considering the size of what most people in their right minds would consider gardens. Anyway, Daddy always had a "garden," he even had a backyard "urban garden" in Florida, and he continued to have one in Colomokee. A few of the local farmers were amazed when he transformed a field full of red sand and rubbish into workable, productive farmland. To his credit, gardening also became a feature of his ministry; he had so much extra produce that he regularly visited "old folks" (whom he often felt were neglected) and took it to them.

Suffice it to say, I knew what picking crops in the Deep South, with gnats-buzzing-into-eyeballs, was like. However, Farm Safety Camp introduced me to the world of modern farm machines. I learned a lot about them at camp, especially that THEY ARE OUT TO KILL YOU!

Really. Trust me when I say that literally every machine on a farm is designed to rip off your limbs and/or spray hydraulic fluid into your eyes. By the time I was a kid, educational institutions had perfected the art of traumatizing children. If I had a dollar for every video I watched of someone dying from AIDS or crack, I wouldn't be writing this book –I'd hire J.K. Rowling to do it. Most of my classmates had to wait a full year to see what skinless human arms looked like, in the "Drunk Driving at Spring Break is Out to Kill You" video series, but not me. I got the full dose early, thanks to Abraham Baldwin Agricultural

College. (Pro TIP: Grabbing a faulty hose on a tractor will result in black, stumpy arms!)

The camp worked, and I never got a job working on a tractor. I did get closer to Summer's family, though-- a much-needed bonus because I was having a really hard time making friends. Unlike Florida, where I had used nonviolent tactics to make friends with some of the people who were picking on me, Georgia was a much tougher environment. First, I looked like Bill Gates. I wore thick glasses, my motor skills were terrible, and I had asthma. Second, I had never really been around a lot of middle-class people before, and their ways were foreign to me. Believe it or not, in the mid-1990s I had never seen a CD player before. (When Summer's brother played a Green Day song for me on his stereo, I asked him to "rewind" it.) My classmates had giant collections of CDs, they skateboarded, and they watched everything on MTV. I hadn't seen MTV in about four years, because we didn't have cable (actually, at that point we had no television at all, because it had been struck by lightning.) I had never owned a computer, and I didn't wear fashionable clothes. In short, I found myself in a culture that was totally foreign to me, made up of kids who had enough money to buy their own culture.

In Florida, my go-to groups of friends had been "nerds," preachers' kids, and "foreigners," while I had grown up around a lot of working-class people in church. None of those groups existed in large numbers at my new school, and my friends from church, like Summer, went to a different school. A few African-American girls were sympathetic toward me (because I was a Christian and they were too) but most of the boys just called me "Forrest Gump" because of my Alabama accent and deepening voice. Meanwhile, the middle-class white kids wouldn't let me into their circle. (I actually mean that, by the way: they literally stood in a circle every day to prevent anyone else from getting in!)

Life was pretty miserable, and I knew that I would have to reinvent myself in order to survive. First, I started hanging around a self-described "redneck." I changed my speech patterns to include lots of unintelligible mumbling and incorrect pronouns. (Summer protested: "Why are you talking that way? You're smart!") This potential friendship was jeopardized after I spent a couple of days unsuccessfully standing outside of the White Kids Circle. I was then rejected by The Redneck, who said "Why don't you go back over there, with all yer high-class friends!?"

After failing at being a redneck, one of my next steps was deciding to remain stupid. No one knew what autism or Asperger Syndrome was when I was in the eighth grade, but I did pick up on the fact that people really didn't like "nerds." I began to purposefully fail assignments, trying to convince everyone that I wasn't very smart after all, even though I had completed a lot of the same work in the previous year in Florida. I tried my hand at being a class clown, and eventually I refused to wear my glasses (at that point, it was more important for people to stop calling me names than it was for me to actually see anything.)

After engaging in the art of pretending to be stupid, my next survival skill was the art of pretending to have money (or at least pretending not to not have it.) For example, with my family bringing in a cool $12,000 per year, and surrounded by the children of teachers and well-to-do farmers, I found ways to disguise the fact that I was eating free lunch at school. I hid the application forms. I got in line last so that no one would see me "pay," or I would enter my number into the computer, acting like I already had money in my lunch account. I also began making strange demands to my mother for designer clothes in an attempt to throw the other students off my trail.

Nonviolence had been an important part of my philosophy during elementary and middle school, but as I progressed through the eighth and ninth grades I began to get into fights. This was partly because I was growing increasingly frustrated with things not getting any better, but also because I didn't want to be thought of as a "good person." Daddy was now pastoring his second church, and for the first time in my life I faced the stigma of being a preacher's son. I didn't really appreciate being pigeonholed that way, so I tried to convince everyone that I was actually a terrible person. After an older boy made an inappropriate remark about Summer, my date to a school dance, I told him to go to Hell and we almost got into a huge fight.

Summer (understandably) never went to another dance with me again. I did, however, keep up the habit of telling people to "go to Hell," "see you in Hell," or basically anything having to do with Hell, because I didn't want to be thought of as "good." When my ninth grade teacher asked us to write a poem about Halloween, I wrote a version of "Up on the Housetop" that involved boys egging houses and then burning in Hell-- because it had Hell in it, and that was bad!

I also read The Outsiders during that time of my life and really internalized it. I was, after all, an outsider. I related to the Greaser characters in the story, and to the violence, too: there was a lot more violence around me than there had been in the past.

I began to lie. This isn't a normal behavior for kids on the autism spectrum, and I was actually pretty terrible at it. Nevertheless, I would tell people anything that I thought would make them leave me alone. If people asked if I was on drugs, I wouldn't deny it, and if people asked if I was going out with Summer, I wouldn't deny that either –it would save me the trouble of being called gay and/or the peer pressure about why I should be having sex with everybody. (I also viewed girls as people, which was something that some of my classmates seemed to have a hard time grasping.) However, once Summer found out about all of this I was in big trouble anyway, and the "lying" phase of my life came to an abrupt halt.

Eventually, I became an atheist (not many eighth-graders I know are making such huge philosophical decisions, shifting from nonviolence to atheism, but I did.) I still went to church because it was next door and my dad was the pastor, but I became fairly antagonistic about it. The best part of my relationship with my father (who had only been a Christian for about five

years) had been talking about God while we were out in the field picking peas. That relationship suffered as a result.

If I had to describe the next couple of years, I would just use the words "dark blahness." While the worst of the bullying stopped after ninth grade (due to older students graduating and leaving town) no relationships with girls were ever working out, and I mostly sat in my room listening to a combination of Nirvana and Delta Blues music. I was chronically depressed, sometimes suicidal.

The Drug Raid

My parents searched my room for the drugs that would have easily explained the state that I was in, even taking away my bedroom door at one point. I responded by hanging a bead curtain at the entrance to my room and buying an old eight-track player with some Led Zeppelin tapes, actions which certainly didn't do much to dispel the myth of drug use. (On the other hand, most people have never had the anachronistic joy of playing Mario 64 to the sounds of Led Zeppelin II, but I did!)

I never used drugs. They were rampant in my school, and some of my classmates tried to sell them to me, but I was never interested, nor did I have the extra money. In retrospect, because of my undiagnosed autism a lot of people's first impression of me was that I must be high on something anyway. I wasn't.

That didn't stop me from being detained during a drug raid at our school, though.

It was wintertime, and there were a few acres of woods next to our house, bordered by a small creek and a beaver dam. I had been hanging out in the woods all weekend, because I thought it was better than having to be around people in the house, and I had taken my prize possession, a red Swiss Army knife, with me.

On Monday morning, with my Swiss Army Knife still in my coat pocket, I went to school. (I may have forgotten it was there, but I also carried it outside of school for protection, due to being under constant fear of attack and/or bullying.) All of a sudden, drug-sniffing dogs (and perhaps a few drug-sniffing police, let's be honest) entered my American Literature class and asked us to line up in the hallway. One girl was strip-searched; in the meantime, two officers with metal-detecting wands came out and asked us to take everything out of our pockets. In horror, I felt my Swiss Army Knife when I reached inside of my pocket, but I took it out and put it in my hand anyway.

At the other end of the line, I noticed The Redneck with a giant Buck knife in his hand. The first police officer (a fellow Redneck-American) walked over to him, admired the giant knife, and went about his merry way. The good-old-boy system had worked its magic! "Whew," I thought. These police officers were after hardened potheads, not people wielding knives, corkscrews, or magnifying glasses.

Suddenly, a cop that everybody called Fats stopped in front of me and looked down at my shiny red knife. He began waving his wand over it: "Beeeep, beeep, beeeeeeep." He looked at it again, and waved his wand again: "beeeep, beeeep, beeeep." Finally, Fats paused, looked at me, and said "What's that?"

"It's a knife," I replied, mildly annoyed but also channeling my best Crocodile Dundee. "Come with me!" he said, and we left the non-criminal element of my classroom behind.

I found myself detained in the front office, sitting next to Violently Sobbing Girlfriend, whose boyfriend had been found to have two seeds of a prohibited plant in his truck. I felt really bad for her, but I didn't know what to say. Besides, I was on the way to jail! The drug arrestees continued piling into the front office, until the police eventually asked me to move into the teachers' mail room to make more room for drug arrests. Within the next hour, all of the detainees were booked, loaded into cars, and headed to jail...except for me, because they completely forgot that I was sitting in the mailroom.

Teachers came in throughout the day to check their mail and ask how I was doing. I told them I was fine. Finally, after 2 PM the assistant principal, Coach Davis, walked into the mailroom, looked up at me, and exclaimed "You're still here?!"

Thanks to a stroke of good luck, I had suddenly graduated, from "drug-detainee" to "school liability problem." Coach Davis took me to the lunchroom, asked the staff to make me a sandwich, and sent me home on the bus. Daddy came by later to pick up my knife; according to Georgia law, a blade under three inches was not considered a weapon.

What is the moral of this story? What can we learn from it? I'm not exactly sure, but consider this: Remember Fats, the police officer who confusedly beeped his wand over my Swiss Army Knife, unnecessarily asking what it was? Remember Fats, who then detained me for having a knife even though it wasn't illegal, then forgot that I was in the mail room when he went to jail?

Fats is now the Sheriff of Early County, Georgia.

Music: My Saving Grace

When I was a kid living in Florida, living away from home for the first time, my parents gave me a shiny red Swiss Army Knife. I was obsessed with them at the time, and after my dad quit his job and went to college it was considered a really expensive gift. It was my most prized possession.

During a drug raid in high school, I was detained for non-questioning due to non-drugs after I forgot to take the knife out of my coat pocket before coming to school on Monday. I carried the knife with me wherever I went.

Tragically, I almost took my own life with it. After years of bullying, failure to "click" with my peers (or communicate with almost anyone) burnout, and depression, I sat alone in my room with the knife in my hand, contemplating the best way to kill myself with it. While I sat, I heard my little sister open the front door of the house. I didn't want her to find me, so I put the knife away and sat back down on the bed.

My saving grace during those early high school years was music. In the eighth grade, I took a music class, playing plastic recorder flutes, and my music teacher Mrs. Helms thought I had a gift for it. She contacted the band director, but I was already two and a half years behind in joining the band. Nevertheless, Mr. Mike Cook, the band director, agreed to teach me if I played the trombone, his native instrument. "Besides," he encouraged me, "trombone players are good kissers!" "Gross," I thought. I learned to play in nine weeks.

At around the same time, I became obsessed with punk rock music. I listened to Green Day repeatedly along with other artists like L7. While it might seem unusual for a kid surrounded by South Georgia farmland to be obsessed with punk, it did give me a sense of individuality. When Green Day sang about disillusionment and lyrics like "...Mom and Dad will never understand, what's happening to me?" I got it. Maybe I didn't understand how I was different from other people, but I knew that nobody understood me. I even shaved my head at one point, but having been hit by a car when I was eleven years old, it turned out that my head was actually pretty ugly.

After surviving the drill-sergeant-like horrors of band camp, I traveled with the marching band and came out of my shell a little. I had the chance to play at the Georgia Dome in Atlanta, and in the Mardi Gras parade at Universal Studios. One day, on the bus, someone gave me some headphones to listen to a song on an album called From the Muddy Banks of the Wishkah. The song was "Smells Like Teen Spirit," and it changed my life, years after the man who wrote it was dead.

I have mixed feelings about Nirvana now. On the one hand, I could relate to Cobain's depression and I learned to play the guitar while listening to his albums. On the other hand, listening to Nirvana so much may have enabled my depression and thoughts of suicide. In any case, I thought it was brilliant, and it fed the "forbidden fruit syndrome" that defined my relationship to rock music.

As a child in the Pentecostal church, I remember hearing some adults talking about a new documentary called *Hell's Bells: The Dangers of Rock N' Roll*. The premise was that rock music was satanic, contained hidden messages, could wilt plants or boil eggs with hellfire-power, etc. (In the filmmaker's defense, the hair-metal of the 80s was kind of evil.) Due to the perception in fundamentalist circles that rock music was evil, I learned to play the guitar in secret. I'm not sure whether my parents would actually have been very critical about it or whether I just perceived things that way, but until my family went over to someone's house and I started playing "Smells Like Teen Spirit" upstairs with their sons, my parents had no idea that I could even play the guitar.

If I had to become obsessed with rock music, I did so at exactly the right time in history. During the 1990s, punk and its radio-friendly cousin "alternative rock" were actually quite popular. The popular kids were actually listening to underground rock music...on purpose! My sudden preoccupation with rock music actually helped to bridge the cultural gulf between myself and the middle class kids. Finally, I made it into the White Kids' Circle (though I still had a stand outside of it for a while first.)

It Gets Better

I started identifying as an atheist at some point during the eighth grade. By the time I was sixteen, I had come to regret that decision, but I really didn't know what to do about it. A generous church member had given me an old 80s computer from a CPA office, which I used to teach myself DOS and BASIC programming. Daddy wasn't very fond of computers, so when someone gave him a hand-held, searchable Bible, he gave it to me, too.

I used to sit in my first period class, searching through a digital version of the King James Bible, trying to make sense of it. To my classmates, I probably seemed like the most hyper-religious person they'd ever met, spending my free time reading a Bible. I wasn't, but I was trying to figure things out. Unfortunately, I just didn't get it. I read every Bible verse as a commandment, trying to figure out how to do the right thing, and trying to figure out how to get back to where I once had been. I tried dabbling in evangelical Christian culture. I got some Contemporary

Christian Music, but most of it seemed to just be pop music with different lyrics; I didn't like very much of it.

That spring, I got a job bagging groceries at a store called Harvey's Supermarket. One of the assistant managers seized on the fact that I was a preacher's son and decided to lay on the Christian-bashing stuff pretty thick. Although I wouldn't have necessarily even considered myself a Christian at that point, I constantly found myself to be the butt of his jokes. For example, the assistant manager (we'll just call him "Bob") would be talking about a song or something, then turn around and say, "Oh that's right, Freddie, you only listen to gospel music!") It was kind of annoying, to say the least.

Bob scheduled me to work on Sunday mornings, perhaps just to be facetious and keep me from going to church. Sometimes I worked until midnight and fell asleep in class the next day, because everyone one else had clocked out and left me with their unfinished tasks. In some cases, when my mom sent me into the store to buy something, Bob would tell me to clock in and go to work.

One fateful day, Bob told me to do something, like usual, but this time he added "and if you don't like it, just turn in your two weeks' notice!" I stopped what I was doing, walked to the counter, and wrote out a notice in the format of a suicide note, ending it with "Goodbye, Cruel World!" The head manager thought it was more hilarious than Bob did.

Suicide jokes aside, as someone who really did struggle with thoughts of suicide as a teenager, I've been pleased to see a video campaign develop in the years since, called It Gets Better. I can honestly report that the campaign's core message is correct: It actually does get better! Over time, the people who made my life miserable in high school simply went away. They graduated and moved on to ruin their own lives and marriages. Some of them died soon afterwards; all of them will die eventually, if you think about it.

Things continued to get better. My friend Summer transferred to my school, and she fit right in with my classmates. I ran for student council, and although I lost miserably in the first round (coming in probably ninth place) I moved up and became a class representative after one of my classmates was suspended and lost her council seat.

Three things happened to me when I was seventeen that were real game-changers. First, after years of not being identified as a gifted student (because I also had an unidentified disability) I was finally put into some honors classes and even early college classes. My schoolwork was no longer cripplingly boring!

Second, I ran for Student Body President...and won! I did have to run against two friends, Bijal, a Hindu girl who was the current vice-president (and only person to ever sign my yearbook) and Michael, an Irish Catholic and fellow trombone player who asked my permission before running. I didn't campaign as hard as Bijal did. My campaign relied on a few gimmicks and some prop comedy. My speech in front of the student body consisted of using a giant pencil to show people how to vote for me, not convincing them why. In the end, thanks to the incoming Freshman class, some outgoing seniors, and a little prop comedy, I won by a plurality of eight votes.

Student Body President = Social Mobility. As the president, I automatically became an honorary member of the local Rotary Club, attending the monthly meetings, eating the golf course food, and being sent to the week-long Rotary Youth Leadership Conference during the summer. In a stroke of good luck, the Mayor of Blakely was also doing a bit of PR before his election, seeking input from younger voters. At the age of seventeen, I was appointed to my first public office: Youth Advisor to the Mayor.

The third (and most important) way that my life got better was spiritual. The week after I returned from the Rotary conference, I went on a mission trip to Central Florida, staying in an old hotel that had been converted into a church. On that trip, I found great meaning in doing things for other people instead of myself. While singing prayers like "I Want to Know You More," I had a profound spiritual experience that would be a defining point in my life. In that old hotel room, I started to not only read the

Bible, but understand it. I began to hum some lyrics from the Live song "Lightning Crashes": "I can feel it, coming back again…"I was on fire, and if I was going to have a new belief system, then I was going to be radical about it.

It had gotten better.

Going to College

From the time I was in middle school, watching reruns of Doogie Howser, I knew that I wanted to go to college. In that time and place, it wasn't something that everyone did. (Of my eight aunts and uncles on my father's side, only the youngest had even graduated from high school.) I wasn't even sure how I might afford to go to college; in my family, the concept of borrowing money didn't really exist.

The desire to go to college had been strengthened by watching my father, who became a Christian and began attending Bible college in Florida when I was about ten years old. He had dropped out of school to work after his own father died in 1979; he had to get a GED before he could go to college.) I saw how hard he studied, and I even sat in class with him sometimes. It was a blessing in disguise that in our household, homework came first, even when I didn't want to do it. My parents, who never really had the chance to graduate, wanted to make sure that I did.

Nevertheless, by March of my senior year I still hadn't applied to any colleges, mostly because I didn't know how. In the meantime, my mother decided to go back to school, to be a special education teacher; every morning, she got up early and drove 72 miles to Georgia Southwestern State University. I finally realized that if I wanted to go to college, I should probably start applying, so I asked her to pick up an application for me. I only applied to one college!

Fortunately, I had a former classmate, a gifted musician named Alvario Smith, who went to GSW before me. He set up an audition with the band director, who also happened to be serving on the scholarship committee that year. Before I knew it, a full scholarship happened.

My friend Summer also went to Georgia Southwestern. In fact, once I moved in, I immediately went to check her dorm out, regrettably forgetting about my parents in the process. When they came back to my room to say goodbye I was gone, so they just went home.

We had a mutual friend from high school named Emily, who offered to pick me up and take me to a magical place called the Baptist Student Union. Unfortunately, I waited in the parking lot and she never came, so I started walking around until I found it. When I went inside, I saw a group of very active people yelling, playing, and doing cartwheels. Their names were Jim, Jennifer, Matt, and John. They were very silly, and they were very scary. They became my best friends.

The Baptist Student Union (later changed to Baptist Campus Ministries, probably because it had the word "union" in it) was a great place to meet people and have fun. We had a flag football team, played a game called Magnum in which everyone was assassinated with waterguns, and even created our own version of "The Mole," for which Jim and I filmed/edited a blooper reel. At that time, there were three Christian groups on campus: Baptist, Methodist, and Presbyterian. In reality, most of the Christian students on campus participated in all three. Nearly all of the friends that I made during college were people that I met at the BSU.

Despite the family atmosphere, outside the walls of the BSU there was a type of legalistic fundamentalism that had been brewing in the Southern Baptist Convention for some time. In 2000, the year that I entered college, the convention issued a new faith statement that prohibited women from being ordained as pastors. Missionaries would be required to sign or otherwise agree with the new statement, so instead of serving as a summer missionary with the Baptists I opted to do work projects with a nondenominational organization, Habitat for Humanity, instead.

Part of the trouble was that the pastor in charge of the Presbyterian Student Center, Deb, was a woman. We all liked Deb, but one night she was invited to speak at the BSU and didn't show up. To our horror, we found out that she had in fact showed up, but that someone in leadership turned her away in tears when they found out she would be speaking about being a pastor. In protest, I joined the local Presbyterian Church. Even though I essentially knew nothing about mainline churches (historically, Baptists had been part of the "Radical Reformation" and eschewed liturgy, the church calendar, symbols, etc.) I eventually became an intern at the Presbyterian Student Center and lived there.

I continued to go to the BSU; the adult leader was a pretty affable guy who had spent his entire career there. As a freshman, I decided to run for the office of BSU president on the platform of bringing in more outsiders. To my surprise, one of the officers came out of the meeting room to tell me "You got it!" and that I was the new president.

For one day.

As it turned out, one of the former officers had come back and expressed her interest in being on board again, so the officers made her president. For the next two years, she headed an organization that had refused to allow female pastors to speak, with no hope of being ordained if she remained a Southern Baptist. In spite of this, she did a remarkable job.

My decision to not be affiliated with the wider Southern Baptist organization, even though my father was a Baptist pastor, was prompted by other events, too. I had grown up around a very diverse group of people. My best friend in middle school was Buddhist, and I attended an interracial church. While I didn't have extremely close friends in high school, the group that I hung around most of the time included atheists, Hindus, and Catholics. I considered it a great thing to be friends with "different" kinds of people, if for no other reason than to be a "good witness" to the Christian faith. I think most of the students at the BSU thought the same way, but there were adults in the community who volunteered at the BSU who began to make executive decisions that suggested otherwise.

One day, I walked out of my dorm and was greeted by a couple of necktie-wearing Mormon missionaries who began propositioning me to join The Church of Jesus Christ of Latter-Day Saints. I told them that I wasn't interested, but that they should join me for lunch at the BSU. We had a great meal, talked for a while, and then they left. I found out later that on their way out of the building, they were actually kicked out, asked never to return.

One event in particular led to a period in my life that I called my "mid-life crisis." I had a friend named Heather who was from a Jewish background. She was (comparatively) short, had long, brown hair, and was part of our close-knit group of friends. Over time we became pretty close, enough so that I called her my "sister."

One dark, humid night, my phone rang. It was Heather, and she was sobbing at the other end of the line. She asked me to come to her room. And as it turned out, an unknown moral crusader had contacted Heather's fiancé in Tennessee to warn him that she was hanging around guys from the BSU too much. I helped Heather pack up all of her belongings so that she could leave school early. She hugged me, said "Thank you," and drove out of the parking lot, headed to Tennessee to save her impending marriage.

I was livid. I felt betrayed. The person who had done this to Heather was presumably one of our friends, and the fact that I didn't know exactly who was responsible weakened some of my friendships at the BSU. Most of my roommates would go on to be officers, and I would occasionally tag along, but after that night I was mentally done. Things would never be the same. Eventually, I started co-hosting a local TV show that filmed on Wednesday nights when the BSU met, and I stopped going.

After being Presbyterian for a little while, I joined a Baptist church that was more moderate, pastored by a woman ordained in a Southern Baptist Church (before the ordination of women was banned.) While nearly all of the best friends that I made in college were people that I met at the BSU, over the course of time I wasn't the only person who was made uncomfortable by the changing atmosphere around the Baptist Student Union. And it wasn't only Baptists who were affected: conservative/liberal purges were taking a toll on nearly all of the Protestant groups throughout the decade. For the time being, at least, it was the moderates who came out on top. Case in point: a few years ago I ran into several of my old friends from the Baptist Student Union at Halloween. As we posed for a picture together, in all of our silly costumes with some of our kids, someone yelled "We're all Methodists now!"

How I Met Your Mother

For the story of the best person that I met in college (after all, I'm biased)...well, I'm going to address this next part to my daughter, who is now three years old:

Dear Miriam,

You are a miracle. It's really that simple. But since you'll really enjoy hearing me blather on about things without rolling a single eye by the time you read this, okay sure. I'll elaborate.

I had a lot of trouble finding a suitable mother for you. In kindergarten, I was all set to marry a girl named Paige, but alas, she was my cousin. (I was encouraged to break off my engagement even though I lived in Alabama. Sometimes people in Alabama do marry their cousins, but you can't.) In the second grade, I liked a girl named Athena... that is, until she ratted on me for being out of my seat. My betrayal at the hands of that backbiting amazon was completely unforgivable!

In the third grade, I met The Most Beautiful Girl in the World, a preacher's daughter named Jessica Jordan. She was my girlfriend for two years, or at least I think she was. I can't really tell because our relationship was a complete secret, actually. We were too shy to talk to each other. I have no idea how we came to the understanding that we were boyfriend/girlfriend, other than the fact that I invited her to my Ninja Turtles birthday party, but it happened.

Just as our relationship was beginning to bloom (i.e. I overheard her actually telling someone that I was her boyfriend) your grandfather, "Tops," decided to go off to college. I was whisked away to a magical world known as the Florida Panhandle, a land where I battled evil monsters known as Palmetto Bugs and bullies. After that, I was too busy slaying monsters, going to the arcade, rollerblading, and reading comics to worry about relationships. (I mean, Superman died! I had to read the comics! It was a time of crisis.)

I did date some girl named Jessica for about a week and she decided that we should "be friends." I don't think we did, though. Angie, the assistant principal's daughter, might have liked me. Maybe not. Either way, I protested a ban on interracial dating at the prom because Angie's mother was being sent away to another school over it. After that, I was hit by a car while riding my bike, and everything got stupid. Then the whole region flooded and I moved away.

After that, none of my relationships lasted longer than about a week. This was not because I didn't like girls (although some people don't, but you can ignore those people. They are called mi·sog·y·nists.) To the contrary, I liked all kinds of girls. I liked girls from Mexico, and Ireland, and Greece, and Japan. I had a thing for Jewish girls, I really liked one African-American girl in my class, and of course, Southern girls are one of the best kinds of girls. But it never worked out. Some of the girls told me that I was like a brother to them, so we couldn't go out because you can't marry your brothers. Some of them said "Let's just be friends." I said "Ok," and then we were friends. I was very polite. I also had good manners, and I was extremely protective of my friends who were girls. But it seemed that I lacked something called "proper social skills," and it never quite worked out.

When I met your Aunt Summer, I thought "Perfect!" and I invited her to a couple of dances. Unfortunately, a high schooler insulted her honor and I told him to go to a very scary place called Hell, where people from high school are tormented and poked with sticks for all of eternity. He refused to go, and we almost got into a fight, which I would have surely lost against such a giant skinhead. Aunt Summer noticed that I was quickly turning into something called "a fool" and so she didn't dance with me anymore. (Besides, when I was in middle school I looked like a weak old man who could barely hold up my glasses and that isn't attractive at all.) I was all frumpy and sad about my fictional marriage with Aunt Summer not working out, but we became good friends. (I married her roommate later on.)

Soon I was in college taking a class called Sociology (or as somebody on Urban Dictionary put it, "the subject of looking into somthing too much." It's really spelled "something.") My professor didn't remember much that happened to him after the 1960s, but he did say there was no such thing as being "in love" because writers from the Renaissance made the whole thing up. Made sense to me.

One night I went with some friends to a house outside of Americus, Georgia to watch a movie. There, among several people I didn't know I met a girl named Emily. She had whitish- blond hair (she was "light-headed," if you will) and back then she looked kind of like a girl from a 1980s movie called The Goonies. Although she was from Americus, the daughter of a local jeweler (whom you call Rocco) she went to school in a town near Florida called Valdosta. We were introduced, but afterwards she completely forgot that I existed. I saw her again at a student conference on the South Carolina border, but unfortunately I was just not memorable enough and she forgot me again.

I liked all kinds of girls, so it would have been simple enough to just choose another mother for you. Unfortunately, the people that I went to college with had never made babies before, and we had no idea what we were doing. One time, during one weird dating experiment, we, the young men and women of the Baptist Student Union just sat in a room and sweated through a series on The Song of Solomon. You don't have to read that book if you don't want to.

Another time, all of the girls I knew started reading a book by a conservative pastor called I Kissed Dating Goodbye. The girls thought this book was fantastic. They didn't need to date! God pointed at me and laughed, saying "HAHAHA!" Meanwhile, an entire generation of Baptists was never born.

Eventually, I got really lonely and started to kind of pray about needing a companion (I didn't want to be "in love," because I learned that there was no such thing.) True, I had companions called "buddies," like Crazy Uncle Jim, or Johnny, or Francisco, or Kevin. But I didn't really want to marry them, and besides, that was against the law before you were born. I had already tried living with them anyway, mainly in unsanitary conditions.

Around that time, I learned that Emily, the girl who didn't know who I was, would soon be transferring to my college and living in my apartment complex. One night, when we were having Game Night at the college, I noticed her across the room. And this time, the third time that we actually met, she noticed me, too!

As luck would have it, I liked to buy shirts from Goodwill. The night that I officially met your mother, I was wearing a fire-engine-red shirt that said "DOTHAN, ALABAMA FIRE DEPARTMENT- JUDGE." I didn't know that fire departments had judges, but all that really mattered was that she saw me playing foursquare and thought that I was a firefighter. And why wouldn't she think that? I played the best game of four square of my life, and we laughed and stuff. That's right, you've finally figured out the truth: my entire relationship with your mother is based on a lie!

Soon we ended up at a lake retreat sponsored by some Presbyterians (we were predestined to be there.) Your mother almost didn't make it because she drove into a ditch trying to follow someone's directions, but finally she did (because it was pre-ordained.) We stayed up all night talking and playing chess and laughing some more.

As predestination would have it, Emily had just moved into an apartment about four doors from mine, and she had already interviewed my friends and roommates. The next night, at her apartment- warming party, we ended up on the same couch trying to dodge a fight between my roommates. I asked her out on my Palm Pilot (it's like a phone but more useless) using a method recognizable to kindergartners everywhere:

DO YOU LIKE ME? ☐ YES ☐ NO

WILL YOU BE MY GIRLFRIND? ☐ YES ☐ NO

She said yes. We didn't get married for a while because I had a job to do, a fearless, important job called "tech support." A new era had dawned in history, and it was my job to make sure that confused, rural people everywhere could get on the Internet. Did the company we contracted with use cheap Canadian technology? Did our customers not listen to our directions because they were beating their children on the other end of the line? Did they call with email questions after unplugging their computers and wiping their noses with them? Yes, yes, and yes! But this job was more important than any trivial thing like "love." And with only one contract, it was far too important for us to be paid in "real money."

After I was laid off and my job was shipped across the border to South Carolina, I got a job teaching. It paid enough real money to buy a ring (except that Emily's dad was a jeweler, so I had to get my courage up in order to buy it from him.) That was really scary, but he was cool with it, so we got married. All of our friends were there...almost. The best man couldn't make it because he was a Marine and had to move to Vermont a few days before. I needed a best man fast...so I chose Summer. We got married, partied, rode away in a trolley and headed to the Caribbean.

The night before I finished writing this story, I had a dream. I was back at move-in day at college and everything was proceeding the same way that it did the first time, except that this time I knew what was going to happen and I could change it. I had more knowledge, I knew myself better, I could really change things, maybe work on some different relationships...

"Nah," I said,

I'll just wait for Emily.

How I Met Jimmy Carter (and the Other Great Man from Plains)

Before I begin, I should preface my story with the fact that yes, I do realize that the words "Jimmy Carter" are controversial. For example, I know that the story of the entire modern conservative movement is based on the fact that Reagan won and Jimmy lost. I further know from experience that whenever I mention Jimmy Carter or post a picture with him for "Throwback Thursday," you might be tempted to say to me, "I sure wish you would tar and feather yourself, set yourself on fire, and go jump in a lake while hanging, you librul!" That's because you, sir, are an Internet troll! If you are a troll, thank you for spending your hard-earned troll currency on this book. You may go back under your bridge for your lunch of horse-leg now, because everyone knows that the Internet is a place for reasonable, nuanced, logical discussion. I mean, people on the Internet carefully consider facts and change their opinions all of the time, right?

Anyway, I'm not stuck in the 1980 campaign and have no dog in the fight because a) dogfighting is very rude behavior, and b) I wasn't alive in 1980 in order to get stuck there. To add insult to injury, I don't even remember Reagan being the President of the United States; I only remember a puppet that looked like him in Genesis' Land of Confusion video. The first, official president that I remember was President Bush; I followed the Gulf War very closely as a kid, because one of my dad's friends from the power plant was sent there and he often called our house from the Persian Gulf at night.

Since Clarke County, Alabama didn't have Internet or trolls in 1991, we had these quaint things made from trees called "books" that we had to get our information from. So it happened that I first heard of Jimmy Carter from a textbook, sitting in Mrs. Kyzar's fourth grade class. It was a very brief description: one term president, Baptist, liked to sit on his porch swing in Plains and drink sweet tea. Other than being president, that paragraph described me! It was a psychologically helpful thing for me, I think, to realize that somebody like me could become the president.

As I grew older and fundamentalists consolidated their control of the Southern Baptist Convention, I started to occasionally see some negative articles about Carter in the Baptist press. Some of the "shocking" headlines (which probably some of the most conservative Baptists would not find objectionable today) were things like "Carter says homosexuals are welcome to come to his church." For the most part, however, he was respected by Southern Baptists when I was growing up. They recognized him as the first "born again" Christian president, who was still teaching Sunday School to tourists every week that he was home.

That was something else that I liked about him: home. No matter where Carter traveled in the world (and he did travel) he always came back home to Plains, Georgia, a small town of 500 people. I liked small towns too, although after my dad became a Christian and subsequently a minister, we traveled around a lot and the concept of home was always a little elusive. Talking to my own family, I discovered that my grandfather Fred Eli Odom, who died in 1979, had been a big Carter supporter.

It's kind of odd, but I basically only remember three things that happened in class during the fourth grade: being moved away from my friend David, telling my girlfriend that I was moving to Florida, and reading a paragraph about Jimmy Carter. Under normal circumstances, I would have read the paragraph and that would have been the end of it, but my life is not composed of normal circumstances.

As it turned out, my father underwent a dramatic religious conversion and the family moved to Florida for Bible college. From there, Daddy became the pastor of a church in Southwest Georgia, where a band director took pity on me and gave me one-on-one trombone lessons even though I was considered too old to begin. Soon after, my mom began commuting over 70 miles each day so that she could go to college in Americus, Georgia. I applied there (because I didn't know how and she could pick up an application form for me) and auditioned for the band. I received a full scholarship, which required a move to Georgia Southwestern State University, a mere ten miles away from the Carters' home in Plains.

At GSW, I went to school with a couple of boys from Plains, along with several other people from Sumter County. One of the Sumter people, a young soldier named Anthony, took me for a drive and showed me around Plains. At the time, he was serving in the army as a Chaplain's Assistant; his unit just called him "Chap Ass" for short. Within a few days of meeting me, old Chap Ass was shipped off to Bosnia-Herzegovina, where I instant-message-corresponded with him for the remainder of his deployment.

Shortly after the departure of "Chap Ass," Jimmy Carter came to speak at the college, and I went to hear him. In a relatively small room, he spoke about his own experiences at the college, shared personal stories, and talked about the importance of the Christian faith in his life. During the question-and-answer session, he fielded a question about Bill Clinton's pardoning of Mark Rich (he simply said "It's disgraceful.") and a question from Anthony's mother Brenda (at this late hour, with my poor judgment, I considered renaming her "Holy Mother of Chap Ass," because that seemed funnier.) Mrs. Brenda's question was simple: "When will my son be home?" Mr. Carter's careful yet honest reply was "The soldiers will probably be there at least as long as your son is there."

I bring up this speech not only because it was my first time seeing Jimmy Carter, but because he made the national news that night. He made the news not for his perfectly decent speech, or for his views on Christian faith, or for his reply to the mother of a soldier. Instead, it went something like this: "JIMMY CARTER CALLS BILL CLINTON 'DISGRACEFUL.' Because the news media were some of the first trolls.

That wasn't my last encounter with the Carters. At graduation my freshman year, the college presented an honorary doctoral degree to Rosalyn Carter. I played in the band, although I was flanked by Secret Service agents, just in case I was a member of a nefarious trick band.

After going to Jimmy Carter's Sunday School class with a group of college students, I visited the church in Plains from time to time. It reminded me of Good Springs Baptist Church, hundreds of miles away back home. I really liked the place and the people; however, there were a couple of obstacles to being more involved there. First, with the exception of people who were already church members, everyone who went to church there had to enter through a side door to be checked out by the Secret Service. I had never been to a church that had church police before, so that was kind of a hassle.

Second, there were the tourists. Maranatha Baptist Church in Plains has a very unique ministry that no other church has. While a lot of churches are doing the best they can to get more people involved, in Plains tour buses literally show up full of people wanting to go to church on purpose, hoping to catch a glimpse of the former president. Personally, I've never been really good at telling the difference between a celebrity and a human, but try telling that to a group of old ladies from New England who believe that they have just seen The Beatles!

Meanwhile, Anthony returned from Bosnia, where he notably talked me out of enlisting after 9/11 and allowed me to meet a friend of his, my future wife. Together, we joined a church that was basically the Carters' sister congregation (but without church police and tourists.) One of the last times I saw Jimmy Carter before I left Americus, he was singing at a Willie Nelson concert. I wrote a music review of it for a Chicago-based site called The Phantom Tollbooth:

"As a rule, I have to respect people like Johnny Cash and Hank Williams. However, I have never really enjoyed modern country music, CMT, or their respective awards shows, which feature Nashvillian suburb-dwellers with giant cowboy hats and boots.

That said, Willie Nelson is one of those huge icons of American music that I can't help but respect, and when word began spreading that he would be giving a free concert in our area, I just had to go. I recalled that Nelson was currently touring the Midwestern states for "Rock Against Bush," but why visit Georgia? (After all, our state has been politically unimportant for at least 10 years.) It turned out that the entire CMT crew was there, complete with flying cameras and "Homecoming" T-shirts.

The logic of CMT's scheme soon became evident: Willie Nelson is from a small town. Likewise, Jimmy Carter is also from a small town. People in Sumter County like Jimmy Carter, like free concerts, and have nothing else to do on Thursday nights. Instantly, a made-for-TV crowd large enough to whiz cameras over would convene outside Plains High School. I arrived with my friend (who shall be renamed "Danthony Avis" to protect his identity) at around 7pm, and we soon located the perfect cloud of smoke from which to view the concert.

The Outlaw did not disappoint. He breezed through all of his classic and most famous songs- "Hello Walls," "On the Road Again," "You Were Always on my Mind," and "Pancho & Lefty," to name a few. His newest hit, "Beer for my Horses" is the type of song that prevents me from being a huge country fan; nevertheless, the delivery by the Outlaw Band was nearly perfect. The highlight of the evening came when Willie brought the Carters on stage, began playing gospel songs, and invited the crowd to sing along.

From my vantage point inside an ever-expanding pillar of smoke, I began observing some of the people standing around me. Some sensed that the concert was coming to a close and took the opportunity to rescue their cars from the parking lot. Others fidgeted or inspected the ground. Still others contributed to my particular smoke cloud without pause. But a final group of people had gleaming eyes, filled with the joy that only gospel songs like "Will the Circle be Unbroken?" or "I'll Fly Away" can bring. And that moment alone made the entire night- even the risk of brown lung disease- well worth the trip that "Danthony" and I made to Plains that night. At the end of the night, the stage was empty and we were finding a shortcut home. As for President Carter- we take it for granted that we'll see him around town again. But seeing Willie Nelson in action was truly a once in a lifetime experience.

[CMT Homecoming: President Jimmy Carter in Plains will air on December 20 at 6:00 PM and throughout the holiday season. CMT is a division of MTV Networks, Inc.]"

Jimmy Carter may not have been history's greatest president. Hearing the stories of my parents who grew up in the 1970s, that decade was hard, inflation was rampant, and every president during the decade (Nixon, Ford, and Carter) left office early. (For the record, Jimmy likes to say that he "voluntarily retired from politics," but it's also true that Reagan beat him soundly.)

I heard a lot about Carter's 1976 campaign in college because my history professor, Dr. Harold Isaacs, literally wrote the book on it. (Meanwhile, I took a lot of his classes, because Dr. Isaacs didn't require us to buy books!) Some of my girlfriend's grandparents had also been part of the Peanut Brigade, a group of grassroots campaigners who traveled to the northeast distributing peanuts and preparing southern-style covered dish dinners for fundraisers. That campaign was remarkable, not only because Carter was the only person from South elected since the Reconstruction period, but because it was entirely grassroots campaign that I don't think would have been possible before or since, due to changing policies and realignment in both parties.

Nevertheless, I mention Jimmy Carter here not because of his presidency or his 1976 campaign, but because he is an example of a role model from Plains who influenced a lot of my thinking on ethics. (If you are a troll, and you don't like that he influenced some of my moral thinking because he's a Democrat, well that's just kind of tough. There is an ogre in your cave stealing your severed goat heads, so you'd better go check on it.)

Jimmy Carter is not the only person from Plains; even if he were, I've only met him in passing. One of my other history professors, a Republican named Dr. Jimmy Bagwell, had lived in Plains his entire life and served on the City Council since 1978. He was a charming fellow who once excused me from class to allow me to cover for another professor, saying that it would be "a great honor." (If you haven't figured it out from Carter's "disgraceful" comment, good Southern men are all about honor!)

Yet there is another great man from Plains, a man that you've likely never heard of but whose story I think deserves to be told. This man didn't have a PhD and he didn't run for President. (He did run, but in marathons.) With a great smile and head full of fuzzy reddish hair, this man was active, full of life, and did everything that he could for others. He was an officer in his Baptist Student Union, and despite his relatively small size, he played in seemingly every intramural sport that the college offered. Like Plains' more famous residents, he was active in all sorts of charities. He encouraged me at a time that I really needed it.

But you've probably never heard of Jay Williams. He died at the age of 31, working at his father's peanut warehouse in Plains. His death was shocking, unexpected. He left behind a beautiful girlfriend whom he planned to marry, and a grieving father who had witnessed the whole accident unfold.

I went back to Plains to honor Jay's life and attend his funeral; my initial reaction that I wrote soon after follows:

"During my first two years of college, before I started filming a TV show on Wednesday nights, I hung out at the

Baptist Student Union, now BCM. While most of the people I knew there are no longer Baptists, most of my really lasting friendships were formed there. On one night in particular, I remember that we took a legal pad and passed sheets around, writing compliments about each other. Jay Williams got my sheet and wrote "Dead sexy."

But he wrote another note on the paper, about genuine faith, that I carried around in my wallet for years. It's likely that I got my first teaching job, met my girlfriend and got married, and moved into our first house with that note in my pocket. Unfortunately, I haven't found it yet since I first heard of Jay's death this weekend."

"Jay's funeral was held at Plains Baptist Church on July 3rd. I have never seen so many people in Plains, or even at a funeral. It was a testament to the life he lived. The streets were lined with cars; I was lucky to find a parking spot at the Lutheran Church. The funeral started at 10 AM, but by 9:40 the church and the overflow room were full. About 60 people crammed into hallways, 20 waited in the basement, and some were outside, including the Secret Service who escorted First Lady Rosalyn Carter. At the graveside service, people parked and walked for half a mile on a rural road, in spite of the heat."

The tributes flowed from all of Jay's friends. Some of them ran marathons in his memory, raising money for St. Jude's hospital. Some offered support to his grieving loved ones. But I think that perhaps the greatest tribute to Jay's memory is this:

This morning, somewhere in Africa, a young mother dipped some water from a fresh well. She leaned over, giving a drink to a small child with pursed lips. In the past, the water made her sick sometimes, but not anymore. There is a new well now. Her child will never know that Jay Williams raised the money for the well, riding a bike across the United States, drinking countless bottles of water that most people took for granted in order to make the trip.

But I do.

As Dr. Bagwell might say, Jay Williams lived with honor.

Koinonia, The Wasp That Killed Me

About a year before I went to college, while doing some service projects in central Florida, I had a Really Big Spiritual Experience (RBSE) that changed my life and made me realize that maybe I shouldn't kill myself after all. My faith (which was mostly nonexistent before, other than my faith in killing myself) became fairly radicalized. I might have even become kind of a zealot for about a month or so. In either case, I know that I leaned in a religious-right sort of direction for a while, because I briefly became interested in Christian media and it was dominated by the religious right: John Hagee, James Dobson, etc.

I carried my newfound enthusiasm with me to college, and I was really interested in finding some Christian peers. (No one in my high school graduating class had been interested in that sort of thing; they were mostly hedonists and quite frankly, a few had gone too far and died as a result.) I made some great friends during my freshman year of college, but I also met some legalistic religious people who ran some of my friends off by being too heavy-handed. By my sophomore year I decided that I really didn't want to be associated with such people, and really didn't want to be labeled a "Christian" at all, opting for the "spiritual but not religious" category instead. To me, religion was something that happened when God wasn't around, and there were really only two commandments to follow: Love God and Love Your Neighbor.

I really wanted to get that second part right and I started looking around for role models. I found several. I read an "autobiography" compiled from Martin Luther King, Jr. speeches, met some local activists, and started to read theology books by people that I wanted to be like. Before it was all said and done I became a humanitarian activist, like a miniature version of Bono, only taller (in fact, I did listen to U2 and even went to three of their shows with my concert buddy Anthony, AKA "the Chap Ass.") At one point, I carried a petition around campus to start a chapter of Amnesty International and I planned to join the Peace Corps after graduation.

Then, September 11 happened, and that disrupted everything. I don't have to describe it. If you were alive in America, you know exactly what you were doing when it happened. I was in the shower in Jordan Hall, and when I came out my roommate was watching the aftermath of the first plane crash on TV. Other than a level of swearing that I have never matched since (which my Pentecostal roommate probably didn't appreciate) my mindset was that we were at war, that this was an emergency, and that I needed to enlist. Anthony, who was serving in the army at the time, talked me out of it (a pretty skillful feat since he was thousands of miles away in Bosnia at the time.) I went to one of the student centers and sat with my friend Micah, while we waited to hear from his sister who worked in the World Trade Center.

From swearing a lot and pledging to surrender myself to the authorities to fight overseas, I kind of ended up in the opposite direction. One of my professors distributed some flyers on campus, on her boyfriend's behalf, about a prayer vigil that one could go to to pray for peace. "What the @$%^&&@&#&@#@#@ &*&@#*&@#&@*#&@," I reasoned. I might as well be doing something. The vigil was at a place outside of town called Koinonia Farm.

I was the only college student who showed up. That night, I tore into the gravel driveway of Koinonia in my beat-up, paint-peeling Chevy Cavalier, listening to some kind of loud, nü-metal music, and asked the first person that I saw "Is this the peace thing?" "Um, yes...this is the peace thing," replied a bearded man very cautiously, carrying a white post. To his surprise, I got out of the car and walked with him, over to a circle of people dedicating a "peace pole."

I didn't understand the ways of some of the people that I met at Koinonia (indeed, it would be over a decade before the word "hipster" would come into common usage in order to describe them.) But I kept coming back, and there was quite an interesting cast of characters there. There was a girl from the U.K. named Victoria, and a man calling himself The Peace Clown, for whom I designed a website. He didn't wear makeup like some of the more scary clowns, he only pledged to wear a red nose and traveled around giving away noses to other people, promoting a message of peace. Geoffrey, the man I met carrying the post, ran a coffee shop in the back.

For some reason, I kept going back to Koinonia Farm. The coffee shop was a quiet place to study during the wintertime, and lunch was always free for visitors (and what college student could pass that up?) The farm was managed by a kindly couple from Illinois named Dave and Ellie Castle. And while I saw Dave as a kind old man who checked on the pecans, there was a lot more to the story. Dave was actually 77 years old at the time, a Yale graduate with a PhD, and a Quaker minister! In short, all sorts of people were drawn to live at the farm. They were drawn there because of a man named Clarence Jordan, who at that time had been dead for over three decades. I came back to Koinonia to take a class about his life and legacy, and his story was a very interesting one.

Clarence Jordan was a Southern Baptist minister who became convinced that segregation was wrong. In 1942, he founded Koinonia Farm as a "demonstration plot," a place where black and white citizens would live and work together on the same farm. As you might imagine, that idea didn't go over very well. The Koinonians were boycotted, shot at, and their produce stands in town were bombed. National guardsmen drove by and fired shots into the building that narrowly missed the children.

Clarence continued working in his shack, translating a version of the Greek New Testament called The Cotton Patch Gospels. It was the Bible in Southern language: Rome became Atlanta, and instead of crucifixion, Jesus died at the hands of a lynch mob.

As the boycotts by the White Citizens Council and others grew more intense, Koinonia might have had to shut its doors (indeed, at one point there were only two families left) if not for Christians in the north who ordered from the farm. And that mail-order business ? It was made possible by a man named Millard Fuller, who despite being a fairly successful mail-order businessman had given up all of his possessions and moved to Koinonia in order to save his marriage.

Realizing that a lot of people in Sumter County lived in old shacks and sharecropper houses, Clarence and Millard concocted a plan to build houses for the working poor without charging them any interest. Clarence would not live to see his dream come to fruition, but under Millard's leadership it would become known as Habitat for Humanity, and when a Sumter County resident suddenly became President of the United States several years later, it went International! The Carters became the face of the organization, working on a house each year for over 30 years.

Koinonia and Habitat were fairly separate organizations by the time I came around, but for a while I was involved in both and saw both sides. As a student in the honors program, I took a class in which we studied how Habitat worked and met most of its leadership. I volunteered making bricks for what would become the Global Village (which comedian Stephen Colbert hilariously skewered as a "poverty theme park" when he came to visit.) Random people came to Americus to give Habitat money; the band Third Day showed up in town once with a free concert and a check for $500,000. I even walked into the Habitat building one day and bumped into the president of Zaire! Eventually, I signed up for a study abroad, working with Habitat for Humanity-Costa Rica.

Living for a short time in another culture was a life changing experience, seeing tropical rainforests, eating fresh bananas, not being able to flush the toilet paper, encountering terrorists...

Well okay, maybe not terrorists. But keep in mind that I went to Central America (where anti-American sentiment is sometimes kind of high because the US government has overthrown the leaders in some areas since the 1940s) the semester after September 11, 2001. We were in the western, less touristy part of the country near the Pacific coast and were called gringos constantly. (I playfully informed them that I was no ordinary gringo; I was, in fact, Super Gringo!) One afternoon, we did encounter a man (I didn't know how to lie and tell people I was Canadian yet) who kept yelling "Yes! Bin Laden is my FRIEND!" My teammate Kirk must have seen the switch go off in my brain, because he held me back and said "Let's just walk away, Freddie, come on, let's walk away...." Kirk is a very wise man. He kept me from being killed and/or being sent to Central American prison that day.

Costa Rica didn't have as huge of a tourist economy and wasn't as much like Hawaii back then. In fact, HOLY CRAP it was dangerous!!! When we first arrived on the gravel runway (they didn't have a big international airport with a KFC then), went to a strip mall to change our money over to Colones. Immediately I noticed a couple of cultural differences. I ordered something from Taco Bell (we were still in the city, obviously) and it had real chicken in it. Also, as we were walking back to our bus someone's car alarm went off and EVERYBODY CARED. Everyone came out of the mall to stare at us and the offending car.

After traveling west for a while, going 70 miles per hour up a gravelly one-lane mountain road on a bouncing bus (because that's normal), and taking a ferry boat, we finally reached our destination on the Nicoya Peninsula, the most dry and mountainous region of the country. I was immediately impressed by Costa Rican culture, because it seemed as though the people there didn't waste anything. Every room in a house or hotel had one light bulb in it, hanging down from a string. Showers didn't have hot water heaters; instead, they were fitted with an electric wire that ran into the showerhead, warming the water slightly. (This contraption was commonly called a "widowmaker," because...well, it's pure electricity running into a showerhead.) This also being my first time in a Catholic country, I noted that there were really a lot of bars. In Clarke County, where I grew up, Prohibition had never been repealed and the sale of alcohol was still illegal. In contrast, the night before we left Nicoya, the Christian family that hosted our team threw a party for us...at their family bar.

We worked on building a house for Don Hermes, a Habitat volunteer who had never been able to afford a home of his own. (In Nicoya, a nice, termite and hurricane-resistant concrete home could be built for around $2,500.) We raised the money before we left by calling alumni; I was tasked with calling a four-star general in Hawaii and waking him up to ask for money. (Not being very fond of verbal abuse, I decided to skip that one.)

Don Hermes had a great family who worked alongside us and they were very grateful. Extremely grateful, in fact: I was a tad surprised when one of his daughters suddenly kissed me. (But hey, you know, those Spanish customs!) One of Don Hermes' daughters came home from work to celebrate both the new house and her quinceañera, meaning that it was fairly normal to live and work away from home at the age of fourteen!

And the food! Such food! There were black beans and rice at every meal, eggs from the yard, pineapple, tamarind juice, and mangoes literally rolling in the street. Several years later someone would write a book about so-called "Blue Zones," which identified Nicoya as one of the major places in the world in which people lived to be over a hundred. While that is certainly true and I did meet a nice old man who was amused by my Super Gringo antics, I dismiss outright the premise that people live longer in Nicoya because of the food. People in Nicoya live longer because they have already survived living in Nicoya, so really, what's going to take them out? They're tough people!

Case in point: there were limited spots available for the study abroad, and all of the guys who were ultimately chosen had former boy scouts. It didn't matter. As gringos, we tried really hard to get ourselves killed. We really did. On the first day, we didn't pace ourselves and became severely dehydrated. As we didn't expect to be so much closer to the Sun, we also burned off a huge amount of our much-needed skin in a short period of time. One girl got sun poisoning and had to be taken to the hospital. Another stepped on a huge scorpion, barefooted. When we went to see the Pacific Ocean, I had to pull a girl out who was getting sucked into an undertow.

Then there were the more alcohol-related dangers. One night, we went out to a karoake club in Carime and I was constantly hit on by a guy who kept trying to get me to dance with him, saying "You daince?" (It wasn't that much of a threat, because he eventually sobered up and walked away.) Later, an unseemly hotel worker attempted to get a girl on our team drunk and take advantage of her. Despite my distaste for/irrational fear of communism, I did what any red-blooded defender of female honor would do: I purchased the biggest Cuban cigar I had ever seen and sat out on the balcony staring at the bastardo. Miraculously, I did not get sick, and after a couple of hours of having a third wheel staring at his face, the man finally went away.

People talk about the culture shock that occurs when they travel to third world or developing countries, but I had culture shock leaving the country. I remember distinctly that on our last day in Nicoya, they fed us Corn Flakes for breakfast, to try to prepare us for acclimation to processed American culture. "I don't want this crap!" I thought. "I want beans and rice!" When we left for the cloud forest of Monteverde to do touristy things, we huddled on the porch of our hotel because it was too cold! "I want my third world room back!" we said. It was strange phenomenon, but we wanted a place where the shopkeepers didn't speak English and didn't accept dollars! We didn't want to leave. When I got home I was inconsolable, and refused to speak English or go outside for a while (because I knew I wouldn't see the mountains when I opened the door.)

In reality, I was probably pretty lucky to have made it back to the U.S. In addition to the other dangers that I listed, I was stung by a tiny black wasp, just two or three centimeters long, on the work site one day. Mind you, I doubt that this wasp was any more poisonous than usual. Maybe the other stresses of the job were getting to me. Nevertheless, I started to hallucinate. Don Hermes walked up to me looking a little worried and asked "Insecto?" At first I answered "Si, insecto!" But then I became delirious and thought it would be hilarious to only speak to Don Hermes in English. Then, when he brought some of my crew to talk to me, I would only speak to them in Spanish! It was a laugh riot!

Meanwhile, I heard a legion of wasps buzzing in the bushes, whispering "Weeer'e commming to get yooouuuuuu..." and thought, "Cool, I'm dying."

Then I passed out.

Christmastime, Living with a Homeless Woman

Early in a December much like this one, I was living in the Presbyterian Student Center (or "Preshouse" as we called it.) I had been offered the chance to be the first male intern in what was mostly a women's ministry, and I gladly took it. For one semester, anyway. Honestly, I had been suspicious of "organized religion," or termed myself "spiritual but not religious," whatever I called it.

People were taking their final exams and leaving town. The place was completely empty and somewhat dark, when I heard someone open the front door. In came an African-American woman, maybe in her thirties, looking for the pastor. I don't remember all of the details, but after she wasn't able to find the pastor, later that night I just invited her to stay. It was pretty obvious that she didn't have anywhere else to go, and after all, I did have an entire house to myself. We ended up living together until around Christmas.

Sheila (that was her name) was very clean; in fact, she possessed more than the average amount of OCD. I offered her food out of my closet, but she never took it. (This was probably due to not wanting to touch it, but keep in mind that I was in college and a meal for me was sometimes just a can of black-eyed peas. I really couldn't blame her.) She typically used the sink to wash herself off, and then spent the day walking around town. She told me that she was originally from Tennessee, but the company she worked for there (pharmaceutical, maybe?) had laid her off. I had literally just found a job myself a week earlier and was training to do Internet tech support. She talked to my girlfriend and me about our future, which we weren't exactly sure about. I was graduating next semester; she had another year.

Meanwhile in church-relations land, the church that supported the student center had a program called "All God's Children," in which we picked kids up from the projects, brought them to dinner, and taught them music lessons. Some of the church members who happened to be from the north (or "Yankees," as people who forgot the Civil War was over sometimes called them) had expressed concern that their kids were around kids from the projects. Just as I was being all adamant in my position that they were just being paranoid parents, one of them asked "where are you from?!" implying that since I was a Southerner (and therefore racist) I should automatically agree with their point of view. This did not help, because a) their implication was stupid, b) "where are you from" is actually a pretty difficult question for me to answer because I haven't decided yet, and c) they were trying to deflect their own racism on to me. I had an "Oh no they didn't!" moment.

Some months later, I was now living with a black woman, in a building that belonged to the church. I'm not sure if exactly the same people were involved, but I started getting pressure almost immediately to kick her out. After some consideration, I decided, "Nah." Now, one might think that a strategy of "nah" could work, but some people are just too darn persistent. Soon one of the best excuses ever used as a trump card followed: insurance. Didn't I know that Sheila wasn't insured to live there? So actually, she wasn't so much a woman without a home as she was a liability! Again, I just kind of failed to listen.

Finally, though, I had to tell her: since she couldn't be in the building when I wasn't there, she would have to leave when I left for Christmas. I wished that I had been more clever and just found a way not to go home for Christmas, but it worked out anyway: when I came back on Christmas day, the heat pump had gone out and it was around 26 degrees (F) in the house. No repairman could be expected to come until after New Year's Day. I found enough firewood outside to last through the first day, before I myself had to live on someone else's couch for a week.

A couple of months went by. I agonized over whether I had done the right thing, or whether I had the right attitude about it. In January, I told the campus pastor that I wanted to be taken off the church's payroll. I didn't mind doing some of the same work for free, but I didn't want the red tape. It would be eight years before I ever did any church work again.

Finally, shortly after Valentine's Day, I checked the mail and found a postcard:

02/18/04

DEAR FREDDIE AND EMILY,

THANK YOU FOR THE HOSPITALITY THAT YOU EXTENDED TO ME.

I SINCERELY APPRECIATE YOUR BENEVOLENCE.

MAY GOD CONTINUE TO BLESS YOU. BEST WISHES FOR A GREAT SECOND SEMESTER IN SCHOOL...

P.S. – YOUR FAVORITE CHRISTIAN BUDDIE FOUND SOME SERENITY! I'M LIVING IN AN INEXPENSIVE LODGE AND APPLYING FOR WORK. IN THE FUTURE, I'LL CALL OR WRITE. TAKE CARE AND BE HAPPY!

FAITHFULLY,

SHEILA

How I Became A Teacher

Recently I wrote a "Who I Am" paper as part of a leadership thing I'm doing at the school where I work. It's not really about who I am, because a real paper about my identity would include my theology (Protestantish), my physiology (mutant), and my favorite music (punk rock). It's more about my outlook on education, or why I teach. Nevertheless, I spent some time writing it (maybe it was a template for this book) and here it is:

"I was born in Grove Hill, Alabama, a very small town in a very rural area between the cities of Mobile, Selma, and Meridian, Mississippi. After my father's dramatic conversion to Christianity and call to the ministry when I was 10 years old, we moved to the Florida Panhandle and later Southwest Georgia. In college, I studied history and political science, met Jimmy Carter and a few other leaders, and worked with several religious groups, including Habitat for Humanity in Costa Rica.

My first trip to Central America was life-changing. In 2005 I went back, and in a village in Belize I discovered that I really enjoyed working with children. I had been getting tired of my job at home, but that problem was soon solved: the Sunday after I returned to the U.S., I was called into a meeting and asked to hand over my keys-- the technical support company that I worked for was closing the next day. Within three weeks of becoming unemployed, I responded to a voicemail from Blakely, Georgia and I was a teacher.

Throughout my life, my educational philosophy was shaped by observing my teachers. Some were good, and some were bad; some were great, and some were terrible. My best teachers thought outside of the box, like the third grade teacher who used a piano to teach Math, the music teachers who took a chance and taught me how to play an instrument in nine weeks, or the science teacher who let me sleep in class because she knew that I had worked until midnight the night before. My favorite teachers were firm but forgiving, and usually pushed the envelope where technology was concerned. Most of all, they loved doing their jobs!

On the other hand, my worst teachers were unimaginative, vindictive, and had probably lost interest in teaching long ago. Some of them were even fortunetellers, predicting that I would go to jail or never amount to anything! These teachers were much more instructive to me than my good teachers, not only because I was determined to survive them and prove them wrong, but also because I was determined not to be like them once I became a teacher. Good teachers should strive to understand why students behave in the ways that they do, have high expectations for their students, and not be afraid to try something new. They should work to ensure that students are prepared for the next grade level, even if that includes college. At the same time, teachers should be careful not to promote the idea that "everyone should go to college" at a time when higher education is in a bubble, the youth unemployment rate is high, and many college graduates find themselves saddled with huge debt and minimum-wage jobs.

If overeducating students solely in unmarketable skills can be detrimental, undereducating students and preparing them all for unskilled-labor jobs (which they'll soon compete with college graduates for) is also detrimental. Career education, character education, and the personal finance skills that we teach in Social Studies are important in avoiding these two pitfalls.

Who am I? I'm a teacher by day, and I tour the South as a performer by night. On weekends I play in a band and teach inmates from a local jail. I'm a new father, a newly elected official, and on some issues quite an activist. When school's out for summer, I can sometimes be found in a quiet corner of Honduras digging a ditch. In other words, I'm a little closer to settling down and answering the question "Who am I?" than I was in high school...and I have the teachers who pushed me (both positively and negatively) to thank for that."

Face to Face With the Ku Klux Klan

One of the things that people who haven't lived in the South very much often wonder about is this: Is everyone there racist?

The answer is fairly easy: No!

However, there is a remnant of good old-fashioned bigotry all over the place, and it never completely goes away. Things weren't always as bad as they are now, or course: they were even worse! To provide some context, less than a year before I was born, in 1981, the last lynching in The United States of America occurred just 70 miles away in Mobile. Some members of the United Klans of America, fresh from leaving a rally, spotted 19-year old Michael Donald walking home from buying a pack of cigarettes. They beat him, slit his throat, and hanged him from a tree in a residential neighborhood (the same neighborhood as an elementary school.)

Despite the terrible fear and grief at the loss of Michael Donald, this time was different. This lynching marked the end of the United Klans after Donald's mother, with help from the Southern Poverty Law Center, sued the Klan. Donald vs. The United Klans of America delivered a $7 million judgment, and Beulah Mae Donald received the keys to all of the United Klans' land and property. I grew up in the first Klan-less society that had ever existed in the South, in the sense that they didn't run things anymore. They didn't even have a place to meet.

Partly because I lived in an area with a huge African-American population, a good portion of what was on TV featured black characters or was syndicated from Chicago. Our local stations aired Fat Albert and a talk show hosted by a woman from Mississippi named Oprah Winfrey. My family gathered around the TV every Thursday night to watch The Cosby Show together... I could really relate to Rudy, when her parents made her stay at the dinner table for hours until the food was gone. Perhaps the most revolutionary thing to me was that I saw black musicians constantly on MTV and VH1: Michael Jackson, his sisters, Lionel Richie, Whitney Houston. I was determined to marry Mariah Carey when I grew up.

My parents were never "prejudiced," as they called it. Daddy was a skilled mechanic, and I remember him going out of his way to help more than one African-American family that was stranded by the road. His parents hadn't been, either. Daddy told me when I was older, "I didn't grow up in a Christian household, but I'm sure glad that I didn't grow up in a racist one."

[Warning: The following story contains mild exaggeration.] Things don't change overnight though, and before all of that happened in my older childhood, my record was far from perfect. Before my uncles were Christians, they were hell-raising teenagers, and in addition to offering me tobacco products at the age of 3, they also taught me the "n-word." One hot afternoon, while my mother was shopping at a Dollar General store, I was running around the store playing with cowboy guns:

"Bang, bang!" I yelled.

"What are you doing?" my mother demanded.

"I'm shootin' me a n-----!" my three-year-old self replied.

Mama, who was born in Europe, was appalled. "I'm so sorry," she apologized to the shocked woman behind the counter, her hands trembling. Were Mama's hands trembling because of shame, I wonder? Worry? Anxiety?

Now that I look back on the moment that almost ended my life, I realize that my mother's hands were trembling due to the "acute stress response," more commonly known as Fight-or-Flight Syndrome. My mama was preparing to fight me with full force, and since I was three years old, I was about to lose!

She dragged me out of the Dollar General store in Jackson, Alabama, beating me every step of the way. Beating and dragging, dragging and beating. Beat! Drag! Slap slap! Beat beat! Drag! Thud! Whack! Thwack! Then she threw me into the car, yelling and slapping. I don't even remember the things that she was yelling, probably about being ashamed of myself. Then Mama drove the car, with me sobbing –SLAP! SLAP! --to Granny's house, where my uncle was still living at home in the back room. She gave my uncle a piece of her mind; I'm surprised she didn't punch him in the throat.

I don't normally advocate violence toward children. In my case, however, it worked like a charm; I became a born-again social reformer at the age of three!

Clarke County's school desegregation order was completed by 1977, and I entered school in 1987. Unlike generations of Southerners before me, I grew up in a completely desegregated environment, or at least I did at school. There were still "white" and "black" neighborhoods around my community of Winn, but I saw them all riding on the school bus. My bus driver was an older African-American man named "Chief," and I spent a lot of time at Chief's house. By "spent a lot of time," I mean that I fell asleep on the bus a lot. Chief would find me during his routine sweeping of the bus after he got home, and call Daddy to come over and pick me up.

My first black teacher was my first grade teacher, Miss Andrews. She was a good teacher, but I mostly remember that she used to hit me with a yardstick or make me stand in the corner and hold up Sears catalogs if I wasn't being still. If that didn't work, I would have to hold a couple of Sears catalogs over my head while standing on one foot! (I'm telling you, corporal punishment was completely normal in Jackson, like drinking a glass of cool water on a hot day. Nobody gave it a second thought!)

Once Mama and I started going to church, at Jackson Pentecostal Church, pastors from black churches occasionally visited and I enjoyed hearing them. Then, when I was in the third or fourth grade, something happened that really disturbed me. On a day that I wasn't riding the bus, we stopped by visit an old lady in town. I went into the backyard and started playing, and a black boy from the neighborhood walked up. We started talking, then running around and playing. We were playing tag or something, when suddenly I heard a booming voice:

"GIT! GIT!

GIT OUTTA HERE, BOY!

GO HOME!"

I looked up and saw the old woman standing on the back porch, waving a broom. The kid looked at me, wide-eyed, and I looked at him. Then he ran away as fast as he could.

"Was he botherin' you?" the woman asked.

"No ma'am!" I said. "We were just playing!"

I didn't fully understand then; I thought maybe she'd just made a mistake. But I understand now.

When I moved to Florida, I had another bus driver named Miss Queen, and unlike any other bus driver I ever had, she played the radio all of the time ("Don't Go Chasing Waterfalls," and "Too Legit 2 Quit") were staples of the early 90s. At the same time, had a sixth-grade teacher named Mrs. Douglas who was every bit as mean as Miss

Queen was sweet, and very frightening. She liked it that way; nobody would mess with her! Fortunately, she liked me because my name was Douglas. She insisted on calling me by my first name, and I didn't argue with her. Together with my sixth grade teachers, Mrs. Douglas asked me to do a presentation on a famous person for the PTA, and they gave me Rosa Parks. To prove to you that I can't make this stuff up, I had to wear a Rosa Parks wig. (I, the white nerdy boy with undiagnosed autism and huge glasses, became Rosa Parks, brave defender of transportation justice!)

One day I arrived at school and all hell had broken loose. Everyone was standing outside, at the front of Graceville Middle/High School, waving stuff around and chanting "HELL NO, WE WON'T GO!" At first I thought these were bad, obnoxious people, because they were saying "hell" a lot and I thought that cursing was probably a sin. Then I heard that the principal had banned an interracial couple from entering the prom. I skipped class and joined the protest. Soon afterwards, I learned that the assistant principal, Mrs. Jordan, had publicly disagreed with the principal and was being moved to a school in another town. Wait a minute...I liked Mrs. Jordan's daughter!

"HECK NO, WE WON'T GO!"

Mrs. Jordan was sent outside to calm us down. She thanked us, but told us that it wasn't necessary and we could go back to class. That didn't work. Then the principal told us that we would receive a grade of zero for every class that we skipped. This bothered me a little, but hey, I had all A's.

The assembled crowd of students left campus to begin the march through town. Suddenly we were surrounded by police cars, lights flashing, cornered in the parking lot of the Piggly Wiggly grocery store. We were forced back across the street, but TV cameras were already rolling. I was in sixth grade, and I learned more that day than I did any day that I was in class!

When I moved to Georgia, it's possible that things were even worse because the area had a history of large landowners who didn't want their kids to go to school with "blacks." When we first moved to Colomokee, in fact, one of the church members, a farmer, offered to pay for me to go to a private school instead (in the Deep South, "private schools" often mean the various "segregation academies" that were founded around 1970.) Daddy refused his offer. For the rest of our time at Colomokee, whenever Daddy preached something that the man disagreed with, he would and pick up Daddy in his pickup truck and take him for "a ride."

Our mailman at Colomokee was an African-American man named Charles Slaton, a friendly, joyful, churchgoing man who brightened up the room around him with his smile. He and Daddy became friends, and when Daddy found out that he was a skilled musician, he invited him to church to play on Sunday night. As Charles began to play, several older men stood up firmly and walked out of the church. "We didn't need them anyway," Daddy said. When Charles died, Daddy went to his church down on a dirt road to preach his funeral. I listened from outside; I couldn't even get in the door.

Most of the people at Colomokee, both young and old, stayed to hear Charles play. They didn't hold such old-fashioned views on race, and even if they had, this was the South: walking out on a guest musician in church was distasteful, and an example of poor manners. The younger generation, even the private school kids, didn't really give it a second thought. We started playing basketball with kids from some of the other churches around our area, and all we really cared about was whether somebody knew how to play basketball, not the color of his skin. Most often, we played in a gym at a church in Edison, Georgia. Unfortunately, when the church found out that a black kid was playing with us, they closed the gym and put a padlock on the door.

These things didn't happen in the 1950s. They happened in the 1990s.

In college, I lived with an African-American woman for a little while (see a previous chapter.) Other than, I lived in a series of dorms and apartments that could get pretty crowded at times, with four or five roommates. When I needed a quiet place to study, I drove ten miles outside of town, to a farm called Koinonia. The farm had been founded in 1942 by a Clarence Jordan, a Southern Baptist minister, as a place where black and white people could live and work together. They were threatened, bombed, shot at. Crosses were burned in front of their property, and during my time going there, there was still a huge flagpole on the property next door, flying a Confederate battle flag.

I had joined a Presbyterian church in response to the Baptists' new policies on women (or specifically, the way that a few Baptists in my town were acting toward them) but I didn't really understand Presbyterianism at the time and I didn't go to church on Sunday very much. I decided to try a Baptist church about a mile away from my new apartment. The pastor, Wendy Joiner, had been ordained by a Southern Baptist church before the practice had been banned, and the story of the church's founding fit right in with my line of thinking.

In the 1970s, the churches in Americus, Georgia posted people at the front of the building. Their purpose: to stop integration of their churches. If African-American churchgoers or "troublemakers" from Koinonia came inside, they were politely asked to leave and escorted out of the building.

A group of people within the church thought that the practice was wrong, and they called for a vote (for readers unfamiliar with Baptist churches, they have a democratic system of government.) Two votes were held. On the first, "Do you think it's wrong to keep people from coming to church?" the majority of the church voted YES. However, on the second vote (whether to stop keeping people from coming to church) the majority voted NO. The members of the church who thought that the practice was an injustice walked out. They formed Fellowship Baptist Church, which I joined right after college. I went there regularly for about four years.

Time passed, I was laid off from my job in a tech support cubicle, and I moved to get a teaching job. I got married, and we borrowed some money to buy a house from my assistant principal, landing us in a town called Bluffton.

One day, I was walking down the sidewalk with a neighbor who had moved to town from Florida and been elected to the city council. Noticing that an old basketball goal in the city park was bent and missing a net, I said "You know, there are grant-writing classes that I can take through the school. Maybe I can look into some money for that." "Oh, we have the money!" he replied gruffly. "But if we fix it those black kids will just come up here and slam on it!" As my jaw dropped, you might realize from my personal history that a revolution was brewing inside of my head. I came home furious, telling my new spouse Emily "We need to do something!"

This emergency was soon interrupted by another local emergency, however, when I walked into school to check my mail. Mrs. Petronia Mike, one of the school librarians, was shaking her head, reading a newspaper and saying "This is terrible." As I looked over her shoulder, I saw the headline:

SOUTH GEORGIA RESIDENTS BRACE FOR KKK RALLY

"Somebody ought to do something," I told her.

But I already knew that that somebody was me.

The rally was being held at the annual Harvest Festival in Donalsonville, Georgia, at the courthouse. Since the town couldn't keep the Klan from using the courthouse, they moved the festival two blocks away, but everything was still going forward. I had no idea what I was going to do and I really didn't know who I could trust. Were some of the local people involved in the Klan?

I thought maybe they were. When I was in high school, my friend Kristen had interviewed some Klan members for our sociology class. There were rumors of a mythical "Goat Man" running around in the woods of Early County, Georgia, and I'd heard it said that the Goat Man was invented to keep children away from the covered bridge at Coheelee Creek, where the Klan used to meet at night.

Not necessarily sure who I could trust at that moment, I wrote to Fellowship Baptist Church asking them to pray about the situation. They wrote back saying that they would, and to let them know how they could help. On Saturday morning, October 18th, I was getting my courage up to go to Donalsonville, when Emily put her hand on my shoulder and said "Whatever you decide, I'm there with you." And that was it. We boarded the car and drove into town. Some of the churches were having a a counter-rally that day, but I didn't agree with that approach and thought that someone who should be opposing them face-to-face.

As I drove around the block, making my final decision about going to the courthouse, our car overheated and I had no choice but to pull over. We walked the rest of the way to the courthouse, where a small group of protesters had already gathered. Even though the Klan was officially protesting illegal immigration and trying to recruit people, the protesters gathered there were mostly the Klan's common enemies: young African-Americans, a gay grocery clerk, a bearded man whose wife was from Mexico. And then there were the two of us, however we might be categorized. On the right side of the street there was a group of Klan supporters, most likely family members.

The Grand Dragon, a beady-eyed, bearded old man, approached the microphone and began to speak. Protesters were shouting, Donalsonville's black churches were rallying, and a hundred miles away, Fellowship Baptist Church was praying. I wasn't kidding about the fact that our car overheated, stranding us at the Klan rally. And just as surely as I didn't make that up, as soon as the Grand Dragon began his speech, the Klan's sound system failed and they were never able to bring it back online. The Grand Dragon couldn't be heard over the sound of the protesters, the media broadcast none of their speech, and they recruited no one. Once in a while they would flip over a banner that read "WHITE POWER" and yell, but other than that everything they spewed was barely audible.

I had come to the Klan rally afraid of what might happen. Now there was nothing to be afraid of. The fact that they actually believed the stuff that they were saying was a little scary, but other than that I actually started to feel a little sorry for them. The local support that I had worried about also wasn't there; a person in the crowd identified one Klansman who worked at a soda factory in Bainbridge, but that was it.

We drove home feeling relieved and victorious. When we got there, there were two dogs lying down next to each other in the front yard, one white and one black. I snapped a picture, thinking it symbolic, and went inside. We sat down and started to get comfortable.

BAM! BAM! BAM!

Suddenly, someone was beating on our front door. I grabbed Emily's hand, then jumped up, fearing the worst. I motioned for her to go to the back of the house, then walked to the front to answer the door.

It was only my neighbor, yelling at me because my dog had run into his yard.

I breathed a sigh of relief, closed the door, and slumped down on the couch.

Remember my neighbor, the city councilman who said that he didn't want black kids playing basketball in our neighborhood? A few years later I was at the city council meeting, signing the paperwork to run for mayor, when he walked in and asked what I was doing. When I told him, he uttered these immortal words:

"WELL, I QUIT!"

Celebrating 10 Years of the GSW Underground!

Nearly ten years ago, I started an underground newspaper at Georgia Southwestern State University, with the help of several friends and roommates. (I would very much like to reprint the first issue for you here, but I think we destroyed all of the evidence.) Since the statute of limitations for making fun of the school has probably passed by now, I will gladly share the story of what happened.

One day I was talking to the campus police chief, Oris Bryant. (Chief Bryant was friendly, he sponsored the African-American Christian association on campus and he was a great barbecue chef, so I liked being around him.) He told me that when he was in school in the seventies, some of the students started an underground newspaper. I thought this was an excellent idea and decided to try it. Unlike the leftist underground newspapers of the 1960s-1980s, however, the ideology of our paper would be satire (something more like The Onion.)

I took the photos from the 2003 GSW news page and altered them, then changed the text around them to create a parody website and paper. (The banner at the top of the paper was the same as the banner at the top of the college website, but with "Underground" spray painted on it.) Under cover of darkness, my friends distributed the papers, putting stacks of them out on racks. I put a URL at the bottom of the paper linking to the web version of it.

I don't remember everything that was in the first issue, but I do slightly remember two things. One of the articles had a photo of Dr. Harold Isaacs, one of my favorite professors. Whereas the original article had been about his Association of Third World Studies, I changed it to an interview using only quotes from his class...and maybe something about how he had been in his office longer than Castro had.

The original "top story," however, had been an article about the college president presenting a portrait to Jimmy Carter, who lived about 10 miles away. In the photo, I put devil horns on the college president's head and changed the title to "Jimmy Carter Meets With Longtime Nemesis Satan." In that story, I recounted how Jimmy Carter, famous for his skills as an arbitrator, had been presiding over peace negotiations with the Devil. There was no mention of the college president's name (although I used his photo-op with Jimmy Carter as the template for my picture.)

Within two months, there was no need to write any more parodies, because the school administration had transformed into a parody of itself. Less than a month after we distributed the first issue, someone gave a copy to the president. In that photocopy, the URL at the bottom was faded, but people in the office reportedly thought that it might have had the word "HATE" in it. Given the evidence that a) I lived in the Presbyterian Student Center, b) the president's picture was changed into a cartoonized devil picture, and c) the Rorschach blot at the bottom looked like "hate" (even though it actually said "Geo Cities") the president allegedly came to what must have been the most obvious conclusion: the newspaper was part of a terrorist plot.

Given the same evidence, dear reader, I am confident that you would have come to the same conclusions; namely, that terrorists were making fun of the school, and that Presbyterians are much like Islamic commandos. If those fantastic conclusions weren't enough, a rumor began to spread that the Campus Police helped to plan all of this. The campus minister also became upset when people also accused her of helping with the paper, so I took the "fall" for everything, reassuring the faculty that I was solely responsible, and that the Presbyterian Church, USA was not a known terrorist organization. In response, I received a letter from the president giving me a word-lashing that I would remember for well over half an hour. Then I burned it in a fireplace. (I am unable to remember or reproduce any of its contents for you today, but I do remember that the tone of it was pretty angry.)

The moral of the story, kids, is this: Free speech is only kind of free, and people in authority do not have the same sense of humor that you and your friends do.

Here's to the tenth anniversary of the GSW Underground's first (and last) issue! I'm really glad that I wasn't taken to live in Guantanamo Bay, and I hope that others will carry the torch, accidentally causing lots of problems by making jokes. I'd like to think that something like the university's reaction couldn't happen today, since almost all media is "underground" now, but you never know.

In the meantime, throughout the president's witch-hunt and in the ten years since, I never admitted that Chief Bryant gave me the idea for an unofficial campus newspaper. Although he did say "You should do an underground newspaper!" I didn't want him to get into any trouble, because he was a great cop and a great person; in Mayberry, he would have fit right in.

Unfortunately, Chief Bryant passed away suddenly in 2013, at the age of sixty. Flags flew at half-staff in his honor.

America's Next Top Model, and How I Became an Actor

There is a movie called *Unbreakable*, about one man who gains superpowers and another who is extremely fragile, his opposite. When you're a person with autism, you are actually both of those people. You have weaknesses, but you gain a couple of extra "mutant powers" as well. You might have great difficulty saying "hi" or making eye contact with someone, answering the phone (or recovering from the sound of the phone) but you also might sometimes speak in equations that baffle people and cause them to look at you like you have three heads. If you speak, that is.

It was such superpowers that landed me my first acting gig, in the Batman Stunt Show. I sat down to watch it at Six Flags, on a school trip, and I immediately started calculating. The man with the microphone took four volunteers from the audience to participate in the show. However, two of the people that he called weren't actually volunteers at all. Two were, and there was a certain pattern to the way that the man picked them.

When the show ended, I stayed in the arena. I moved to the center, slightly toward the front, away from the rest of the crowd, and waited for the next show. In the next round, I was picked almost immediately, thanks to a little pattern recognition.

Unlike the fake volunteers who served as hostages in one of the fight scenes, my objective was fairly easy: to party at Wayne Manor. And party I did! I had to wear a tux, dance with a pretty Filipino woman in a red dress, and not step over a certain chalk line in order to avoid being hit in the head by clowns on motorcycles. Stuff was exploding all over the place! Finally, Batman zip-lined across the arena to save the day, defeating every last one of the clown motorcyclists!

That particular trip to Six Flags happened because I was in the marching band; I also got a full scholarship because of it. When I first showed up for band practice in college, I saw a sight that made me burst into laughter. There was a man, sitting and leaning on a cane on one side of the room, watching us practice. And it just so happened that this particular man, other than being thin and gaunt, looked exactly like KFC's very own Colonel Sanders!

This was no colonel, however. This was Claude Speer, a fellow who had once worked at the college as a maintenance man until he retired in 1978. He was around eighty years old, had never married, and had very little family. However, instead of sitting around the house all day, as was his right, he came to every event at the college that he could... provided that it started after 11:00. ("It's taking longer for me to get out of the house," he told me.) He was at every band practice and concert, every baseball game, and he went to First Baptist Church every Sunday. He literally knew hundreds of college students, past and present, by name. I often ate lunch with him and listened to his stories of life at the college in the 50s, 60s, and 70s. (He had particular disdain for one college president he'd worked for, never failing to remind me that "He was a smart ass!")

Claude Speer, being eighty years old, gave me two pieces of sage advice:

1) "Education is a back-stabbing business!"

He told me this when he found out that I had considered adding on a teacher certification. He was right about education, of course. I had already noticed this trait in high school.

2) "You have a good stage voice."

I'd sung when I was a child once, but I was otherwise deathly afraid of crowds until I got older. Eventually, he was proven right and I was indeed spending my nights on stage.

It happened thusly: shortly after we got married, Emily found out that a Methodist minister she knew as a teenager was going to be moving to our area. While he had served in Peru for a number of years, his family was finally moving back to Georgia after someone tried to abduct their twin sons. Shortly after arriving in Colquitt, Georgia he invited us to go with him on a trip to Costa Rica. I had enjoyed my time in Costa Rica before, and we had never been on a trip like this together, so we decided to go.

Several people from Brother David's church went, and it proved to be a life-changing experience for a lot of people. In particular, there was a big, red-haired man with a hearty laugh and a goatee named Chuck. Chuck had brought the whole family along, and after this particular trip he decided that he wanted to live there. He gave up his industrial cleaning business and moved the family to "the Mayamundo," Central America. I visited Chuck and his family in Honduras and Costa Rica after that.

Perhaps due to Miller County, Georgia's history of Irish-ness, there were several people on our trip notable for having bright, red hair-- something that the people in Central America had never seen. One particular red-haired person caught my eye, though, a hippy-looking girl of seventeen or eighteen. She reminded me of someone I knew in high school whose life didn't turn out so well, so I decided to have a talk with her and lay some advice on the table. To my surprise, she kind of appreciated it.

Her name was Tarah, and she was the daughter of the music director for a production called Swamp Gravy, the official play of the state of Georgia. She had been an actress for roughly fifteen years, and she, along with Chuck's son-in-law Lee, invited me to to play in a band that they were about to put together. Eventually, our band played once a week for jail inmates who were attending a recovery program.

Not being in actual recovery (or actual jail) ourselves, Lee and I often went to this dive bar called The Powerline (literally named that because the only other thing on the property was an electric power line.) We ate lunch there on Sundays with some friends, because no matter what diseases might be present in the building, the food was delicious.

Walking out of the Powerline one day, a man stopped me and said "My daughter would like to talk to you!" I nervously followed him back inside. Of course, my first thought was to respond "Sorry sir, I'm married," because I assumed that men in Georgia must be so impressed by my Victorian-Era, trained-by-old-people manners that they would immediately consider me to court their daughters.

Instead, it turned out that The Man's daughter, a girl named Victoria, had seen me playing the guitar earlier in the day. Having seen this, she must have reasoned "This guy does stuff in front of people," and she invited me to audition for a play that she had written called Sister Queens.

"Will it be fun?" I asked.

Victoria and her mother, who was sitting nearby, were taken aback by this question. They responded:

"Um, sure!"

"Okay," I said.

The next night, I drove 40 miles to audition for the play. (Victoria and her mother later told me that they never in a million years thought that I'd actually show up .) I read some lines, and then Victoria said "Ok, do you have a song?"

"What?!"

"Can you sing a song?"

I thought fast, but not fast enough, and then I just started singing a Bob Dylan song. It was probably fairly terrible. But Victoria was in such a hurry, and she needed someone so badly to fill a part, that she conceded to my demands that the show be fun. I landed the part of "Donny," a character originally intended to be the middle-aged MC of a beauty pageant gone wrong. Instead, I played a character who was the younger, extremely manic, dysfunctional and ambiguously gay MC of a beauty pageant gone wrong.

Seeing how much of the cast was composed of teenage pageant girls (and men pretending to be teenage pageant girls) there was more than a little backstage drama, complete with clashing egos and/or personality disorders. But I didn't care. Fun was guaranteed in my contract, and I meant to have it. The show was a smashing success, breaking some previous records for the Olive Theatre. Unbeknownst to me at the time, Mr. Claude Speer (the man who had first encouraged me to use my stage voice) died while we were rehearsing the show.

After all of the cast-partying and the run of the show was over, I stayed in touch with the cast of Sister Queens. (After all, my modus operandi has been to have mostly female friends, and then to be irrationally protective of them.) We got together one more time for a DVD release party before going our separate ways. Some of the girls went off to college. Two of the cast members, Will and Susanne, were also a part of the cast of Swamp Gravy and they went back to performing in that show. (Will eventually went on to work for Disney Theatrical Productions, and when he was chosen to write Swamp Gravy's 20th anniversary show, one of the stories from this book, that of the interracial prom protest, made it into the show in edited form.)

Victoria continued acting and modeling. As with the other girls, I wrote her a note of encouragement now and then. Eventually, Victoria's modeling led to two consequences:

1) An April Fool's joke titled "Weekend With the Models," in which I posted photos of myself allegedly hanging out with models, wearing stupid hats and a bandana photoshopped to read "CoExist."

While the execution of this April Fool's Joke was flawless, it didn't actually work because when people saw it, they just kind of said "Makes sense." and moved on. A few women did become very angry with me, however, for allegedly leaving my wife to hang out with models all weekend.

2) Victoria became 15-minute famous!

Victoria's real name is Victoria Henley, a contestant on cycle 19 of America's Next Top Model. I won't comment much on the contents of the show, because honestly I was disappointed in the way that she was treated and portrayed. I was also disappointed that (perhaps due to non-disclosure agreements) Victoria's dad was never mentioned on the show. In real life, he's a great guy, a veterinarian and a founder of the recovery program that our band played in. Victoria was portrayed in the show as being joined at the hip with her mother and very dependent, but her dad was never mentioned.

I sent Victoria some notes during the filming of the show, but she wasn't able to respond to them until afterwards (due to the aforementioned non-disclosure agreements.) Sensing that she could use some positive press, I wrote a blog post of support that went semi-viral, though I see no need to quote it here. To her credit, Victoria has survived and used her TV persona to launch a career teaching workshops to kids. She called me "bold" once, and I wore it as a compliment.

Randomly, Victoria called me up a few months ago to film something with Miss Teen Arizona for a film festival. I went, fun was still in my contract, and that's all that I can really say about that right now. Maybe it will see the light of day.

After initially working with Victoria, I helped some friends with a children's acting camp, and they encouraged me to try out for this show called Swamp Gravy. (The show is based on true stories and is named after a local dish that makes use of all sorts of ingredients, much like the people in the show.) When tryout time rolled around again, my friend Tarah (whom I met in Costa Rica) called and sealed the deal. I auditioned and became a part of the Swamp Gravy cast. Within the next year, I had toured and performed the show for over eleven thousand people. (Not too shabby, for an introvert.)

The next year, I had to step up my game a little and play ten roles, in a show about about the murals in town (the Global Mural Conference, because it exists, was held there that year, and we performed for it.)

The characters I played in that show were:

-angry citizen

-street preacher

-shopkeeper

-Jack, a "good-for-nothing" character who gets his car battery repossessed

-a moviegoer

-Elvis Presley in a cafe

-Jailhouse Rock Elvis

-One of the Anglin Brothers (escapees from Alcatraz) dressed as an old woman

-firefighter

-returning WWII soldier

That meant a lot of costume changes (whew!) but it was a lot of fun (again, fun is in my contract.) And while impersonating Elvis was great, I also ad-libbed quite a bit with my street preacher character (I told the director, Jerry Stropnicky, that I was "putting the "fun" back in fundamentalism.") I created one-line sermons for him, and before the run was over I had covered each of the Seven Deadly Sins, among other things.

ON GLUTTONY: "You gluttons are pushing my buttons!"

ON LUST: "When He finds out you lusted, you're gonna be busted!"

ON ENVY/GREED: "Keeping up with the Joneses will put DEBT in your boneses!"

ON GRADUATION: [for graduating seniors] "When you pass grade twelve, don't wind up in Hell!"

ON CHARLIE SHEEN (more or less): "You call it winning... but mister, I call it sinning!"

ON GHOSTBUSTERS: "Dogs and cats, living together...mass hysteria!"

You get the point.

One thing that I was not prepared for when I joined the cast was a weird celebrity effect that occurs only once a year, when students from Florida State University come to see the show and attend a conference about it. Having been told all weekend that Swamp Gravy was groundbreaking and great and famous, I sometimes find myself strangely hit on (or even hit) by some of the female students. It all happens like this:

1. The people who attend the conference are there to learn about how great Swamp Gravy is, and how to be successful in their own hometowns. They basically already know about and like the show before we perform it.

2. I am the only male in the 18-30 age demographic performing in the show.

3. I attend the conference, and end up in the same room as all of the people who watched the show and want to be more like Swamp Gravy.

4. Therefore, I spend the weekend beating FSU girls away with a stick (not literally though, that would be terrible behavior.)

The first time I did the show, this weird behavior was unexpected. One girl hit me and ran away giggling. She hit me! By the end of the weekend, I had deputized Susanne as my official "bodyguard," and I surrounded myself with people that I knew, especially at mealtimes. It was a winning strategy. The second time, I didn't stay for the conference (but I was still cornered after the show by a girl named Hiba and went out for Chinese with her friends. No problem there: I like patrons and food.)

By the third time I did the conference (and attended it) things had gotten a little weird. After the show, one woman wouldn't let go of my hand after shaking it. At 9 AM the next morning, conference-organizer Robin asked me to help a girl set up some recycling bins, making us late for class. The girl, Esther, asked if she could follow me to class "Sure," I said, and started getting into the car.

"You're driving?!" she asked.

"Shouldn't we be protecting the environment?" she asked.

I walked to class with Esther.

Once we were in class, the speakers encouraged everyone to leave their tables and find someone they didn't know. Who did everyone suddenly not know? Me! I suddenly found myself in a group with at least two girls from Miami. At dinner, new designated bodyguards and friends of the show Kendra and Tarah witnessed a woman walking past me, waving in my face, and shouting "Howdy!" (Howdy? Kendra said she "squeaked.") I walked into the parking lot where another girl waved at me really fast and talked about the show last night.

Finally, I sat down to watch the storytelling cabaret that a group in the conference put together, sitting safely with friends. The seats directly in front of and behind me magically filled up with FSU students. After the cabaret, the audience was asked to group with cast members to discuss something, and I found myself in a large female-only group. A woman kept asking me to say things so that she could hear my accent.

Don't get me wrong; I like the FSU students very much. Those girls are out to change the world, and I hope that they do. I'm also glad that I only have groupies once a year.

Our cast has had a lot of great times together and I could probably tell a lot of stories about them, of going on tour, and of what we jokingly call "Swamp Gravy: After Dark." I'm not going to do that. Instead, I'm going to share just one story, the one that is my favorite, the one that is the strangest, the one that I titled "THEY COME FROM TOWN!"

"There is a guy named Smitty, a big-hearted, big-bearded fellow who's in the show with us this season...except that he wasn't in the show at all last night. You see, Smitty has launched a career as a DJ, and he had a gig at a club out in the country last night. After the show, a few of us decided to go out and pay Smitty a visit, to encourage him in his new chosen career path.

Before we went, we stopped by White's Bridge so our costume designer could scare some ghost-hunting teenage girls. (Libby, a young woman playing a ghost bride in the show, jumped out of the woods and chased them.) Then we drove up to the place (just down the road,) looked at the bare aluminum building for a minute, and walked inside. The inside looked a lot like my uncle's garage, plywood with a rebel flag and pin-up girls on the wall, probably advertising beer. One key difference: my uncle's garage does not have A STRIPPER POLE in the front of it! Once we got inside, my friend Susanne turned to me and yelled "FAIL!"

She wasn't the only one yelling over the music, because as soon as we walked in several guys at the bar in the front of the garage looked at us and started yelling (in succession) "They come from taown!" "They come from taown!"

They were trying to intimidate us. It worked. Having now designated the bar as a scary zombie place, and not wanting to dance around the pole, we decided to go to the very back of the building, close to Smitty, and play off our fears by playing darts instead (I won't lie, I did take a picture with the pole.) Unfortunately, I threw the darts like I was playing tennis, and mainly just broke a lot of darts.

By that time, it was about 1 AM. Smitty was packing up his equipment and we no longer had an excuse to hide behind the sound table. We decided to run for it. If you've ever seen the "Bob's Country Bunker" scene from the movie Blues Brothers, you understand what it was like. Mean-looking redneck people, confused looks, spinning tires.

I haven't been to another one of Smitty's gigs yet."

Letters for Emily (No Relation)

I have previously:

a) written that I am exceedingly protective of my female friends, and

b) brought up the fact that I made several new ones in the course of performing/filming "Sister Queens." For the most part, I have kept up with those cast members and tried to offer support when possible: a babysitting job here and there, a supportive letter when they're on America's Next Top Model...you know, the usual stuff. I did invite one girl, Sierra, to Swamp Gravy and ask her to come up on stage with me for the "Hoochie Coochie Dance," so she basically owes me nothing now.

One of the girls in Sister Queens was still in high school when we met, and when she found herself in times of trouble, I used my god-like powers of...well, not being in high school anymore, to offer support and write letters threatening anyone who might mess with her. In the first letter, I explained that Emily Cloninger was from Tennessee, where she was considered royalty, and recommended that the bully instead bow before her. With permission, I have reprinted the second letter, which I gave her to carry around school in case of emergency, below:

Dear _____:

This is getting ridiculous. (Maybe even redonkulous.) I hope that you are not one of the same people that I wrote this letter to last time, because if you are, I am getting the lunchlady to hide something in your sandwich. What is your least favorite thing to find on a sandwich? Raw chicken feet? Pickled horse nostril? The cockroach, perhaps?

Soon you will find yourself eating "a triple-decker sauerkraut-and-toadstool sandwich with arsenic sauce," if you do not comply. Did I not warn you to appease Emily (who is royalty) with tiny gifts? Let me define tiny gifts for you:

Marshmallows are tiny. But miniature marshmallows are TOO tiny! Why would they make a miniature version of a food that's already tiny?! Do not be led astray. For example, if you must appease her with a diamond ring, remember that rings are only tiny versions of bracelets, and get the diamond bracelet instead. But remember that a diamond hula hoop is too big.

Speaking of too big...aren't you in high school now? You are acting like you have no sense! I would understand if you were in the eighth grade, but once you get into the ninth grade you should start looking for sense! Because if you don't have it, things end up in your sandwich! Grow up, you crackhead, or I will destroy you!

Signed,

Shiva, Destroyer of Worlds

As you can see, I take all of the credit for Emily graduating from high school. Eventually, she began her college education, like all royal highnesses do. And in college, she struggled with a brand new nemesis, the accursed Algebra! I had no choice but to write a threatening letter to it as well:

Open Letter to Algebra:

Dear Algebra:

It has come to my attention that you are giving Emily a hard time. I must quote the Beatles when I say: "Get back to where you once belonged!"

Yes, it's true that you control all of the bridge-builders and computer programmers and a few scientists, but it's high time the rest of us throw off your harsh rule. We history teachers, Waffle House cooks, farmworkers, writers, plumbers, electricians, factory workers, heavy-machinery operators, tech support-ers, actors and musicians simply do not need you. Small business managers don't need you, and large business managers keep algebrists on staff anyway.

Simple business math is sufficient for most people, if not basic math. And cashiers don't even need to know basic math anymore, thanks to microchips. The main group of people who DO need algebra? The guild of math teachers at colleges, who would have to find some other job if they didn't require students to take algebra. Many of these students who are good at math already realize that college might be a bad investment anyway.

What do you have to hide? Why do you cover up AMOUNTS with LETTERS? That alone proves that you are not trustworthy. My digital clock and bathroom scale are both more honest than you. Even Dairy Queen tells me the EXACT amount of calories in my chili cheese dog!

Yes, Algebra. Your rule is coming to an inevitable end. Hardly anyone needs you anymore. The microchips and "Texas Instruments" that you created have made you unnecessary. The only reason we still talk about you is because of something called "laws," whereby people can be made to pay for unnecessary things by force (like copyright laws forcing people to buy "Get Back" when anyone with a computer can now make their own copy of the song for free.) If states didn't require your class, you would already be living in exile.

For now, Emily will take your class and meet your requirements. Nevertheless, Algebra, you had better sleep with one eye open. Like the people before you who pumped gas, picked out cotton seeds, washed clothes on a washboard, copied books by hand in monasteries, or put on toothpaste caps in Charlie and the Chocolate factory, you are about to find that your job is no longer required."

To Emily: sorry I haven't written you a letter in a while. I hope you can settle for this book instead!

Oh, THAT Phillip?! My Chance Meeting With an American Idol Winner

I have met a few celebrities in my life, some before they were celebrities. I don't tend to get all excited about it, because I do sometimes have a hard time telling the difference between a celebrity and a person.

The first celebrity I ever met, after playing in the high school marching band at Universal Studios, was actor Kevin Sorbo, of TV's *Hercules* and *Andromeda*, and of Movies' "films with stereotypical atheist professors in them." I was walking around with two girls whom I kind of liked (I couldn't decide which one I liked better) when suddenly, who should appear before us but Kevin Sorbo himself, dressed in the garb of the demigod Hercules! The girls that I was with became giddy, and they lobbed their cameras at me just as surely as they lobbed themselves at Kevin Sorbo. I dutifully took a photo of the three of them.

"HA HA HA!" said Kevin Sorbo. "They're really making you WORK!"

"@#*#@#!# KEVIN SORBO," said my jealous brain. [In fact, I will now officially go on record as saying "Screw you, Kevin Sorbo!"]

After the boom of reality television, I met a couple of the stars of reality TV. I've already written about Victoria, but there is another.

From my blog, May 27, 2012:

"I haven't watched American Idol since maybe 2006, but all year I've been hearing that there was some "kid" from Leesburg named Phillip Phillips on the show. Recently, I wrote on this blog that even though I hadn't watched the show, I'd be glad to vote for Phillip Phillips, and wished him the best of success, whoever he was. Phillips won, after a mind-blowing 132 million votes were cast [on American Idol]...more votes than are cast in a presidential election. This weekend I was in Gainesville, Georgia to be a groomsman in my friend Anthony's wedding. {Long time readers of this book should remember that Anthony's nickname from the army is "Chap-Ass."}

We went out to Wild Wing Cafe, where I think the waitress was a little disappointed that none of us actually ordered food (eating a rehearsal dinner tends to spoil your appetite.) Anyway, after the usual Braves talk, we got on the subject of American Idol, and Phillip Phillips. Someone asked, "Don't you know him, Anthony?" Anthony answered in the affirmative and started describing him, then stopped and said "You've met him too, Freddie!"

"Oh, that Phillip?!"
Not having watched a single clip of American Idol this year [or in ten years] I never stopped to realize that I knew who Phillip Phillips was. I just called him "Phillip" because I always had trouble remembering his last name. (Yes, really.) So here's the story:

Phillip's sister LaDonna and her husband, both missionaries in Jamaica, founded an organization in Albany, Georgia called Mission: Change to fight homelessness. I took part in one of their rallies a couple of years ago, called "Sleep Out for the Homeless and Hungry," where people basically spent a cold night in front of the Albany Mall sleeping in cardboard boxes. There were a few speakers: a pastor and a member of his church who until just recently had been homeless, and the director of the local Habitat for Humanity chapter.

There was also a band playing...a pretty good band, in fact, led by a guy named Phillip. Anthony introduced me to the whole family that night, and I kept bringing up Phillip in conversation from time to time because a) I was really impressed by the band, being something of a musician myself, and b) the band played Michael Jackson's "Thriller." This stuck in my memory, both because it was awesome, and because I've never heard another live band play it before or since.

Lo and behold, according to Wikipedia he second song that Phillip played during the Idol auditions was... an acoustic version of "Thriller."

It's a small world after all."

Why Late Isn't Great (Book Edition Bonus!)

After I finished the Kindle Edition of this book, I was digging around in my parents' house one day and found the Holy Grail of things I have written, a handwritten essay called "Late Isn't Great." I wrote it when I was fifteen to explain why I didn't pick up my uniform from the cleaners. (The real reason was that my family didn't have eight dollars, but who wants to admit that?) My band director, Mr. Ferry, commanded that I write a four-page essay explaining why my uniform was late. I subsequently tried to fill up four pages with as many words of teenage angst as possible, as well as whatever was currently airing on *Channel One News.*

A couple of things to understand moving forward: "Buzz" was Mr. Ferry's dog, and Jimmie Murkerson was the sheriff. Also, a widely mocked profile sketch of the Unabomber circulated in the 1990s.

And now, without further adieu...

Late Isn't Great

Part I:

Why My Uniform Was Obviously Delayed in its Safe Return to the Early County High School Band Room Even Though I Am the Most Dedicated Band Member I Know Who Is Not Conceited, Pregnant, or Currently Partaking in Some Form of Substance Abuse or Just Sitting There Staring Into Space Because of Stupidity

by Freddie Odom

This is the title page*

* title page- (tītal pāj) – n. - a single page containing the title of one or more essays, reports, legal documents, etc. Most title pages are usually comprised of a title, personal information such as the author's name, teacher and/or date. Most title pages are white, but informal title pages may be various colors, such as blue, red, purple, green, orange, brown, pink, fuscia, black, yellow, magenta, or any other shade of color produced by the Crayola company.

Before I begin, I would like to in-form you that the reason my uniform was returned late is because of the weather phenomenon known as El Niño. It has provided a number of setbacks, the first of which was Bill Clinton stealing my uniform to pick up women. After receiving the Con-gressional Medal of Honor for beating him up and stealing my uniform, I hijacked Air Force One and crashed violently in the Pacific Ocean, where I spent the night chatting with Gilligan, Skipper, the Millionaire, his Wife, the Movie Star, the Professor, and Mary Anne on Gilligan's Isle. That morning, lo and behold, who should come by but Lassie on a raft. I bid the natives goodbye and cruised into the school just in time. Hearing a harsh voice, I whirled around to face Aunt Bea from the Andy Griffith show!!!

But alas, it was only Mrs. Drew. She sent me to the office for thorough drug testing because she said I vaguely looked like Judy Garland. On my way to the office I was attacked by savage Norsemen on a journey to find Elvis Presley, who proceeded to carry me out to their camp. I was surprised to find that the Vikings had with them a dog named Buzzz!

Part II:

How Buzzz Wuzzz and How I Believe the Wind Ensemble Should Be Called the Elite Band Forever Hereafter

After a long fifteen minutes in the Vikings' camp in the pressbox, I decided it was time for Buzzz and I to escape. I signaled Buzzz. He rolled over, fast asleep. "Forget Buzzz!", I exclaimed, and began running for my life. The Vikings tripped and fell down.

That evening, the doorbell rang. I opened the door to find a man with sunglasses wearing a hooded jacket. "Here," he said, handing me a brown parcel. He began jogging down the road with Jimmy Murkerson behind him. (Perhaps he wanted to have donuts and coffee with the jogger.) I set the package down on my uniform, thinking "That's really nice of that swell chap!" Then it exploded, blasting one button off the uniform and out of the window. Then I ate some strawberries from Mexico that were tainted with E. Coli and vomited on the uniform. If frantically mounted Mr. Ed (who was a horse, of course) and rode to the cleaners. By the time I brought the uniform to school the next morning, however, it was too late.

Part III:

The Beginning of My Insomnia and How I Neglected to Mention That It Was All Fred's Fault.

My uniform had arrived too late. The Great Dave, after throwing down and having an A Natural fit, decreed that I should stay up until the wee hours of the morning writing this true account of why my uniform was late. This is okay with me, because I have learned to forgive Dave.

My heart will go on.

Part IV: The Charges Against King Dave

I. He has struck his head repeatedly against the chalkboard.

II. He has oppressed and threatened our people with voodoo sacrifice

poles.

III. He has established ten commandments not of the Bible.

IV. He has actually put up with BOB.

V. He has inscribed exploding heads on the same board on which he hit his

own head.

VI. He occasionally insults one's mother using mental telepathy.

For these transgressions we shall do absolutely nothing... because he was

paid to do this and can readily withdraw us from the Early County High

School Band if he wishes to do so.

The End

The Chapter That Will Get Me Fired

As of this writing, I'm about to begin my second term as a mayor. After I finish writing it, I may not be elected to anything ever again. But it's okay, I value time off.

Several years ago I co-hosted a TV show on the Americus/Albany GA public access channel called The Student View. Unlike Crossfire or other shows at the time that usually featured Democrats and Republicans yelling in one another's faces, we jokingly opened with this:

"On the left, I'm Chesley _____!
...And on the OTHER LEFT I'm Freddie Odom!"

Then we'd play an opening song like "Rubber Band Man" or "Soul Bossa Nova."

The producer, Genie, was a friend of mine and had originally invited me as a guest before asking if I would help host it. Our crew consisted of a guy from Louisiana named Matt and a Frenchman named Oliver. (Indeed, there was something French about the whole thing.)

I constantly made fun of how low-budget our show was.

One time I decided to turn around and show the audience that the skyline behind us was actually just a green screen, because there were, in fact, no skylines in rural Southwest Georgia.

Shortly after joining the show, I found out that my beautiful co-host Chesley had a girlfriend. Most people didn't know. I figured it out in the course of hanging out with her; sometimes the cast and crew went out for Mexican food after filming the show. (I had so little money that I often just ate chips and drank water because it was free. Ah, simpler times.)

I hadn't known anyone who was openly gay before coming to college. In fact, on any given day on the radio, driving to school, I heard very alarmist stuff about gays destroying the fabric of America and bringing about DOOM! When I saw a gay rights activist signing people up for something at my dorm my freshman year, I just kind of nervously walked past her and walked away to my room.

In fact, I was kind of "homophobic," not in the actual sense of hating gay people, but in the literal word-meaning sense of being scared of gays. I mean, they were trying to destroy America and everything. My college band director was gay, and when I auditioned for the band and found out that I would have to be in a room alone with him...OH NO!!!

Finally, when I went to Costa Rica to do work for Habitat for Humanity, I roomed with a gay man who taught at the college. But you know what? He didn't randomly attack me at all. He wasn't a rainbow-throwing terrorist! He was just an Episcopalian. With some friends from school, I took a couple of trips to The Monastery of the Holy Spirit in Conyers, Georgia. There, I saw a young Catholic monk who had chosen a life of celibacy, because he was gay.

Back at the television studio, as I looked across the room where Chesley and her girlfriend sat, the veil was lifted for a moment. Who was I to want to boss this girl around, or be afraid of her? We weren't that different (like me, she was the child of a Southern Baptist pastor. Also, I liked girls too.) At that moment I had a revelation of sorts, and I saw that she was perfectly human, she was perfectly beautiful, and I loved her.

It's a good thing that I thought that. Because several minutes later, Chesley sat next to me in front of the camera, went off-script, and announced to the world that she was gay. (I just sat there looking stupid, because hey: you go off-script with an autistic person and it's like taking a key and locking up their brains. I got better, though.)

Here's the thing: if you're a Christian and you use the literal method of interpreting Scripture, then you probably see homosexuality as a sin. If you tend to use the historical method, you probably don't. There are a whole host of other positions in between. But that's neither my concern nor my area of expertise.

For Christians, whether you see gays as your neighbors or your enemies, Jesus didn't make a distinction for you. He said "Love your neighbor" and he said "Love your enemies." If gay rights activists don't understand the Christian faith because they only see a caricature of it on TV, that's not their fault. It's yours and mine.

For people with autism, our perspective is a little different, not only because we're less likely to make distinctions between people, but also because some of our experiences are similar. I was bullied as a kid, I was called a "sissy" because of my smaller size and a "faggot" when I didn't have a girlfriend. Besides, there is reason that autistic people have borrowed the term "coming out." If you receive your autism diagnosis as an adult, it's a relief to know why you're different from other people. It's hard to tell your friends and family, but it's a relief when you finally do. And it's disappointing that when people finally find out, some of them change their behavior and treat you like a leper.

There is a common issue on which I think everyone can work together, and it is this: the suicide rate among autistic teens is a staggering two percent. 1 out of 50. (This is personal to me, as I was almost one of those statistics.) The suicide risk among gay teens, while not quite as high, is about five times greater than the general population. Shall we guess what the staggering rate among autistic gay teens must be?

One of the only times I've ever used social media for productive purposes (i.e. not clicking "like" on photos of cats) was just after college, when I used it to raise money for a girl from North Georgia. She was kicked out of the house after coming out to her parents; I raised money so that she could buy books for school.

Was I "enabling her lifestyle?" Would she have been better off if she had dropped out instead? I don't know. What would Jesus do?

The One About Me "Coming Out"

As for me, I was diagnosed with a mild form of autism in my late twenties. Everything that had happened to me in the past started to make a little more sense, but I was a little worried about telling people. I had been on the city council in my town for less than a year, and I worried that people would think that I was less capable of doing my job (which I had already been doing for several years anyway.) Soon, however, I picked up a copy of a regional magazine called Southwest Georgia Living, and it just so happened that two of the features that month were 1) a feature on Swamp Gravy, with a photo of me on stage, and 2) a positive profile of some people with autism who lived in our region. I thought "Maybe the time is right." Besides, I was tired of having to be careful about who knew and who didn't.

On February 29, 2012 I wrote a post explaining my decision to my blog readers and supporters. As far as I can tell, I was the first elected official in the U.S. to publicly identify as autistic, although I looked for others and would be happy to hear from others. My original post is below:

"Imagine that you were born with a series of genetic mutations that gave you some pretty cool abilities: super-senses, super-memory, the ability to create and maintain worlds, or the ability to predict almost anything with mathematical certainty. These abilities would be apparent at a pretty early age. With superior vocabulary and math skills, academics would be a piece of cake. Maybe you would ponder ways to skip a few grades and be like Doogie Howser.

Having these abilities would come at a cost, however. As someone who is vastly "different," you would spend your formative years as a social outcast. After all, while your peers are learning how to throw a football, you want to learn how to build robots. Sometimes, you're completely oblivious to the opposite sex, and on the odd chance that you're interested in someone they're oblivious to you. You're perfectly happy with most of your friends being girls anyway, and the rest of them seem a tad immature.

Meanwhile, you're stuck in an institution called "school," where you are grouped with others solely based on age. This is bad, because people your own age know something is up. Your teachers really don't appreciate it if you correct their math or spelling, either. To survive the trial by fire that is public school, you decide that if you're going to blend in with regular humans, you're going to have to ditch the glasses and play dumb. Learn to act like a class clown (after all, a well-played joke can deflect a punch) and learn to play the guitar (unlike your computer programming, it's something that you can do in public.) Survive long enough, and you can filter out some of your less desirable peers by going to college early to study something less boring to you.

As you get older, you try searching the Internet to find out what makes you different. No luck. Native American or Jewish ancestry? Maybe you were adopted, or crashed from another planet or something. After all, you do seem to relate better to K-Pax, or Superman, or Spock. What does God think about all of this? You'd like to know the answers, but there are other pressing matters. The world is unjust anyway, and you want to do something about it.

Finally, you start to find out that there are others like you. They have some of the same abilities and have had some of the same experiences. Most of them are also in their twenties, trying to figure it all out...maybe tens of thousands of them, even. Around the same time, you hear stories of people trying to find a "cure." In France, they are using electroshock therapy. An executive in the U.S. has a grandson with the mutation who is unable to speak, and so the executive begins a crusade. Finding a cure becomes a nationwide, sexy cause, and billions of dollars are raised, even by toy stores.

If there was a cure, would you take it? If there was a genetic test, would future people like you be aborted?

If the above story sounds like a plot from a science fiction movie, it probably has been before. But it's also the story of my life, one facet of it anyway.

My name is Freddie Odom, wearer of many hats, and I am autistic. I decided to tell everyone in the March/April issue of *Southwest Georgia Living*, and now I think I'll just sit around and wait for the backlash. Be nice in your comments; remember, an autistic person probably designed the screen that you're reading this on!"

Mayor...Here Comes the Internet!

Initially, there wasn't much of a backlash after all... at least not until I became Mayor a year later. Then came the trolls, and this is how it happened:

First, a little background. I have tried all sorts of political philosophies, and "found them wanting." I was a Democrat in the second grade (because that's what Southerners did) then I was a card-carrying Republican from the age of seventeen until the invasion of Iraq in 2003. I donated my high school wages to the campaign of George W. Bush and Dick Cheney. However, after the war began I really disagreed with that decision and I became an independent (until the present day, even.) College Republicans invited me to their meetings. College Democrats invited me to their meetings. I never could seem to find the time.

At first, considering that Republicans were wrong because of the war in Iraq and having somewhat rigid thinking, I thought that the opposite must be true: maybe liberal Democrats are completely right! I joined an online forum made up of democrats. I had a session on there called "Ask an Evangelical Dude," in which Democrats could ask me questions about what being an evangelical was like. I hoped to correct some of their misconceptions about it, because they were blaming Christians for everything that Bush ever did wrong. But before long, I realized that a good many of the people on the site were just as uncivil, extreme, and hateful as any other political group on the Internet. I left. Perhaps ironically, I left the forums at Christianity.com for much the same reason, and I was much happier with fewer trolls around.

By 2007, I was working on a Master's degree in military history and trending toward libertarianism (in America, a libertarian is basically an anti-war conservative, but sometimes also socially liberal.) I kept my old usernames, because I liked to read more than one point of view before making a reasonable decision about something. (You know, what people always do on the Internet!) I used my former political knowledge to start putting together collections of public-domain political speeches, some from

Republicans, some from Democrats-- whatever I thought people might be interested in buying.

After I became mayor, however, I made a critical error in judgment. I went to the Democratic forum to tell the people I knew in the past that I had become a mayor, and to ask if there happened to be anyone there who had done any work with disability rights. This was a huge mistake for two reasons:

1) People on the Internet started defining my ideology for me:

"Well, it's NICE to have a REAL PROGRESSIVE in Georgia!" was one example. I was even congratulated by a user called "Egalitarian Thug." (?!)

2) People on the Internet sit in front of computers all day in order to dehumanize their enemies and fling excrement at one another.

Every day of the year, there are political hacks who read one another's websites all day, looking for attack fodder that they can use for character assassination. When I posted on the old democratic forum to say "Hey guys, update, I'm a mayor now," the neoconservative members of another forum went into internal war panic, saying to themselves "OH NO! THEY ELECTED ONE OF THEM!!!"

They started trying to dig up stuff on me. They found the Swamp Gravy YouTube channel, and called the city clerk. They made fun of my neighbors, calling them stupid, disabled, or generally just made fun of them for living in rural America.

Did I go to their website to try to talk it out? Did I say, "See you guys, there has been a misunderstanding and I'm probably more conservative than you on _____ issue, and anyway I don't really participate in your level of politics because like the Mennonites I think..." Heck no, I didn't! One does not simply feed the trolls of the Internet!

They went on to make brilliant autism-related comments:

"What a place! No one filed for mayor except the town nut."

"He can add to his collection of prescription bottles full of hair clippings..." etc. etc.

Oh well, C'est la Vie.

They can kill me, but they can't eat me.

On Politics

The field of politics is sometimes ironic or amusing. Take, for example, this gift that someone gave me once, of Rush Limbaugh Sweet Tea. The slogan is "from tea to shining tea." To me, it's funny. To trolls and extremists, it is deadly serious.

Sometimes politics is dangerous, such as in the case of every war, ever. But most of the time, in my daily life, politics is just plain boring. Whenever the latest political issue arises, I ignore it. Sometimes I don't vote. While politics was a hobby for me (when I was a political science minor) and I even had a TV show dedicated to the topic, I am supremely bored with it. People have told me that I am apathetic. I want to reply "No, I'm just better at math than you."

I may or may not be better at math than someone else. What I mean is that it is very predictable to me. I have successfully predicted every presidential election since I started paying attention to presidential elections. In 2008, I wrote the editor of an electoral vote prediction website telling him that he was wrong about Omaha, Nebraska. He disagreed, but I turned out to be right.

In 2010, someone asked me if I would put a sign for a Republican candidate in my yard. Problem: there has never been a Republican congressman in my district (unless there was during Reconstruction) and the Democratic candidate was going to win. After the hardest, most passionate, and most expensive campaign ever waged by the GOP in my region, the Democratic candidate won by 10,000 votes. Not 10, mind you, ten thousand! I was correct in not wasting my time and energy. By the same token, if a Democratic candidate comes through my neighborhood running for Senate, I'll ask him what his plans are when the campaign is over, because he's most likely going to lose (a "she" might have a better chance of winning, but not likely.) During the political cycle, I will mostly ignore what all of the candidates say. At best, I'll sometimes watch shows on Comedy Central that mock the political process. And I'll be much happier. As Thomas Jefferson once said, "I do not take a single newspaper, nor read one a month, and I feel myself infinitely the happier for it."

That said, all politics are local, and there are things that every person can do locally to make a difference. Blowing hot air in a debate sponsored by General Electric at a presidential library somewhere doesn't make a difference to hardly anyone, except for advertisers.

What, then, can the average person do? Well, they could do something, anything, instead of considering their neighbors the scum of the earth and attacking them all of the time. One may find this hard to believe, but sitting around waiting to vote for someone every four years, then grabbing one another's throats in between the votes, is not the best way to solve problems. And it isn't meaningful to anybody.

Try this: Are you against abortion? Support crisis pregnancy counseling and adoption. Are you against war? Support Christian Peacemaker Teams. Poverty? Volunteer for the Salvation Army or a soup kitchen. Homelessness? Build a Habitat house. Anything that you can do yourself (or with your group) will work 100 percent more efficiently than your request for a politician to get something done.

As for my own party affiliation, when I was running for mayor I held a mock campaign online to raise money for St. Jude's hospital (in honor of Jay Williams, whom you might remember from "the greatest man from Plains.") One of my mock campaign promises had been "to join a third party in order to make them feel better about themselves." I did, and I joined the Libertarian Party for a year (as they're the only registered third party in my state.)

I don't necessarily agree with them either, and it's my preference to just remain independent for the time being. That may come as a disappointment to some people, but it shouldn't. There are causes you can support, movements that you can join directly, and things that you can take care of yourselves. And if you do it right, you'll never be alone.

My personal heroes are people like Dorothy Day, or Clarence Jordan, or Millard Fuller, who started movements and worked to solve problems from the ground up. I don't think we're necessarily much different than them.

The world needs activists, and the world does need radicals. As Larry Norman put it, "We Need a Lot More Jesus and a Little Less Rock N' Roll."

But mostly, the world just needs you. You're all that you have to give, and you're enough.

Afterword: A Surprise Ending

If I might take the liberty of blowing the ending to our show, Swamp Gravy, it usually ends with the song Amazing Grace. Candles are lit, and the cast members call out the names of the people in the community, including former cast members, who have gone before them, saying "I remember you." Most often, I call out the names of two of my students who have died: Ricky Cardenas, who died in an accident, and Garrett Justice, who was shot by his own father. It might be the only way that they're ever remembered.

In some small measure, I hope that is what I've said to my friends, family, and mentors with this book: "I remember you." On one level, I wrote it because my grandmother died, and for my daughter and younger cousins who will come after me, facing some of the same struggles that I did. On yet another level, I was just trying to reinterpret my life in light of the fact that I'd been struggling with a form of autism the whole time and just never knew what it was called.

In August 2012, I needed to take a test to become the certified water system operator for my town. I decided to go to Mobile, Alabama to take the test, so I could stop by and visit some family members. Since other people who took the test before me complained about the math questions, I went to Granny's house, as I had done for twenty years, to study. ("Study hard and make me proud!" she always said.) I'm glad that I did, because it was the last time that I saw her alive in her own house. Granny passed away on February 14, Valentine's Day, 2013. I wrote this account of her passing about a month later:

"Last night, we were reading my daughter a story and I sat down on her bed. I immediately smelled my grandmother's house (we stayed there a few weeks ago and took Millee's pillow with us.) I was pretty useless after that, so I just went to bed. I've been trying to stay busy and avoid thinking about it since she died three weeks ago. It's how I deal with things.

It's not that I'm necessarily sad that Granny is gone; to the contrary, I never really spent a lot of time thinking about

Heaven very much until the past few weeks. During her last year, she enjoyed reading stories about near-death experiences, and actually had been preparing to go for quite some time. Last year, I gave her a copy of Nearing Home by Billy Graham, after one of my tennis players' grandmother let me borrow hers.

Still, we were pretty close. I made the trip to see her as often as I could, although she was quick to remind me that I didn't call her as much as Moriya did (another cousin, who uses phones.)

My Granny, Margie Vice, was born in Marengo County, Alabama during the Great Depression. Her mother died at an early age, her father remarried, and her new stepmother basically put all the children out on the street; they split up and lived with relatives in other towns.

She married Fred Eli Odom and raised nine children. When his health started to fail in the 1970s (and he eventually died in 1979) she went to college at the age of 50 to become a nurse. She retired in the 1990s, and in 2001 she contracted Guillain-Barre Syndrome from a flu shot. She never completely regained movement in her hands, although she had previously sewn her own clothes during most of her life. For another 12 years, her doctors marveled at the fact that she was still alive...her diaphragm wasn't working! Nevertheless, she continued to teach Sunday school every week, until life on an oxygen tank made her less mobile and Good Springs Baptist Church closed last year.

A lot of people would say that Granny had a hard life and never had very much. But on the night that she died, there were representatives from all nine branches of her family sitting beside her. She loved Southern Gospel music, and the women sang songs, like "When We All Get to Heaven":

When we all get to heaven,
What a day of rejoicing that will be!
When we all see Jesus,
We'll sing and shout the victory!

Everyone was cheering her on and telling her that it would be ok, she didn't have to fight any more. My daughter Millee said and waved goodbye, and while there were a lot of tears in the room, people were also at peace about it I think. She passed away at 11 PM central time, on Valentine's Day. The family stayed with her body for several more hours until the funeral home took her from the hospital. On the following Sunday, all of her grandsons united for the first time, as pallbearers.

Granny never believed that would be the end of the story..."

My impossible life would never have turned out the way that it did if it weren't for my father, Fred Odom, who converted quite suddenly to Christianity and was called to preach by the time I was ten years old. I never met his father, who died of a heart attack on July 4, 1979. Daddy always told me that he was kind of a hard man, and he had never told him that he loved him. As a conservative Baptist,

I think the possibility that his Daddy might not be in Heaven haunted him throughout his early preaching career.

As I was finishing up this book, my parents moved in with me while the house that they were living in was being remodeled. We celebrated Daddy's 54th birthday. When I came home from work one afternoon, Daddy looked at me and said "Well, Freddie, you might get to meet my Daddy after all." I was a little confused, and taken aback, not quite sure what I'd just heard. Daddy sat down on the couch, tears welling up in his eyes.

He'd been talking on the phone with his brother Bill. They had a long conversation about a lot of things, but Bill told him one story that he had never heard before.

Just before their Daddy died, the children were clearing off the land around the house that they lived in, in Winn. They cleared it off by hand; with nine children, they did everything by hand: gardening and hunting, fishing and fur trapping.

Their daddy, Fred Eli, was suffering from a previous heart attack; only 20 percent of his heart was really functioning. He often stopped to rest, sitting on a pine stump halfway up the hill, getting sap all over his clothes. One day he went outside and went to the stump by himself. When he came back, he told everyone standing there that everything was going to be alright. The Lord had spoken to him, he knew that he was going to die, and everything was going to be fine.

In the 35 years since his father died, Daddy had never heard that story. Maybe it would have changed things if he did. But I can't help but wonder what else God told my grandfather that day. Maybe he knew some of the things that were going to happen in this book.

Fred Eli Odom.

Marjorie Vice Odom, "Granny."

Aunt Anita. Aunt Kathie.

Miss Lena Reeves, "Mee Maw."

Flaudie Bradford.

Nettie Nall.

Shirley Finney.

Elige Steadham.

Bicey Elizabeth Taylor, the baby.

Mr. Mike Cook.

Jay Williams.

Dave Castle.

Millard Fuller.

Oris Bryant, "Chief."

Claude Speer.

I remember you.

See you soon.

THEY CAN KILL ME

Freddie Odom

BUT THEY CAN'T EAT ME

Made in the USA
Lexington, KY
19 October 2015